RISE *and* THRIVE

A mental health workbook for youth & for the young person inside all of us

A guide to intentional caring for your mental health

By Dr. Alfiee Breland-Noble

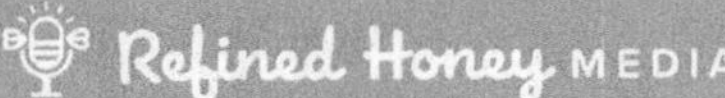

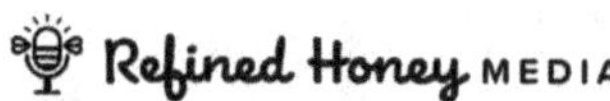

Arlington, Virginia

Contact Us:
dralfiee.com
MGMT@dralfiee.com

ISBNs: 979-8-9939236-0-4 (hardcover); 979-8-9939236-1-1 (paperback); 979-8-9939236-2-8 (ebook)

Illustrations courtesy of Down the Street
Book design by Mayfly

Library of Congress Catalog Number: 2025924014
First Printing 2026

To you, Gran, because they sent you into the swamp but could not hold you there.

To you, Mama Alice, because NO weapon formed against you could prosper.

For you, Grandmother, because you are a trailblazer,
leaning on the everlasting arm.

And for you, Mama, because I love you—my road dog—
those pots and pans have plenty of dents.

To Miss Hattie at the Fuquay-Varina Super Walmart: This is for you,
because yes, we have come a long way.

For my Day . . . remember, the emperor has no clothes, but he's got an R01.

And to my soulstar and the comets, Dr. Richard and the M&Ms. I adore you.

Contents

Introduction

***Rise and Thrive: A Mental Health Workbook for Youth and for the Young
Person Inside All of Us*** is the culmination of my life's work—both profes-
sionally and personally. I wrote this book *for you,* to help you feel seen,
heard, and valued, especially in a world that often pushes marginalized
young people, like People of Color, LGBTQAI+, and those with disabilities,
to the sidelines.

As a Woman of Color and a mental-health professional, I want you to
know: *I've been where you are.* I understand what it feels like to navigate
spaces where you don't feel fully accepted or valued. I've been the only
Person of Color in a room, the one person who doesn't quite fit in, and the
one who's been made to feel like I don't belong. And it sucks. *But,* that's
why I'm here to walk beside you, to remind you that *you're not alone.*

I can vividly remember the life-changing incidents that fueled my drive
to help others. My earliest memory is of my brother. I was in fourth grade
and he was in third. He was the sweetest soul, a gentle giant who stood
taller than most of the kids in the entire grade. Unfortunately, he had a
racist teacher who was very unkind to him. He was one of only two Black
children in the class, and he often came home and told us about her negative
attitudes toward him: She would single him out for behaviors that multiple
kids were engaged in, she made rude comments about his size compared to
the other kids, and she would often not call on him when he raised his hand
in class. He was asked to stay after school with her one day for "tutoring,"
so I took it upon myself, unbeknownst to our parents, to stay with him. I
sat in the hallway and asked her to keep the door open. She was angry that I
was there and was rude and laughed at me after she interrogated my reasons
for being there. Even as a ten-year-old, I understood racism, cruelty, and
injustice when I saw it. I felt compelled to help, even if all I could do was be
a witness. Needless to say, my keeping watch helped my brother and put the
brakes on his teacher's cruelty—at least for that afternoon.

This is how I have been throughout my life—a champion for those of us
who have ever felt underappreciated, unseen, and unheard. In high school,

I became the first president of the Black Student Union. Then, in college, at my beloved HBCU, Howard University, I volunteered for the PEACH (Promoting Educational and Cultural Health) program, which was designed to train Black college students to mentor some of the most under-resourced, talented, and promising youth in Washington, D.C.

In graduate school at New York University, I volunteered as a youth afterschool program mentor at University Settlement, a settlement house for Asian (mostly Chinese) and Latino (mostly Dominican and Puerto Rican) recently immigrated and transplanted kids and families. Then at the University of Wisconsin, Madison, I mentored racially diverse student athletes, helping them transition into the university environment. This thread of addressing disparities, pushing for equitable outcomes, and being a champion for young people's mental health continued in my time as a young professional, when I was one of the first people to write about and seek to address the needs of middle-class Black youth with depression. This culminated in my creating The AAKOMA Project in 1999 and transforming it into my research lab at the Duke School of Medicine, where I earned my fourth and final degree.

While at Duke, I was a scientist in academic medicine (which is essentially the educational and research side of medicine), dedicated to centering and uplifting the mental-health needs of racially and culturally diverse youth through community collaborations with young people, their families, and their communities. All of this was grounded in the research that we generated, together.

I share all this with you because personal and professional experiences are the fertile soil used to germinate this book. I've included practical, accessible resources throughout this workbook—which is meant to be interactive and fun, not some dry textbook you'll never open again. This book is for you to pick up, put down, flip through, laugh with, and maybe even cry through. You'll find video drop-ins with me (yep, I'm *that* personal) and exercises to help you get rooted in and connected to the person who matters most: you! It's my goal to help you feel supported, uplifted, and empowered every single day, no matter what you're going through.

We all stand on the shoulders of giants, which is easy to forget in this culture where it's all about the "hustle" and the "grind." But here's the deal: *None of us get anywhere alone.* When you hold a marginalized identity, there's incredible strength in standing behind yourself—uplifting yourself, supporting yourself, and finding tools that help you thrive. This book is one of those tools.

Yes, connecting with your community is important and powerful. But before you can do that fully, you need a strong foundation within yourself. I wrote *Rise and Thrive* as the permission slip that lets you focus on you—your needs, your growth, and your mental health. Because everyone deserves a space where they can feel safe, valued, and supported. Too many young people don't have that kind of space, and I know that the world often sends harmful messages that make you question if you belong. If you've ever felt like you don't quite fit in, like you've been fighting for your seat at the table, I want this book to be a safe place for you—a warm voice reminding you: *You belong—and we need you!*

Be Your Authentic Self—No Holds Barred

One of the most important lessons I want you to take from this book is that embracing all of who you are is an act of courage and power. I'm not talking about the "Instagram-perfect" version of yourself—I'm talking about the *real* you. The one who's a work in progress, the one who's still figuring things out, and the one who's constantly evolving. When you start by understanding yourself, giving yourself care and compassion, and prioritizing your wellness, you create a ripple effect. You help others feel safe to do the same. You create a world where everyone has space to shine, and there's room for all of us to thrive.

A question I'll help you answer in this book is: How do I show up as my authentic self everywhere I go? For many of us with marginalized identities, society sends us constant messages that there's something wrong with us. Let me be clear: *There is absolutely nothing wrong with you.* Those messages don't even come from you—they come from people and systems that are uncomfortable with your brilliance.

I know it can feel overwhelming at times, especially when the world seems like a hostile place. It's easy to wonder: *Where do I belong?* The truth is, figuring out where you belong starts with building a strong connection to yourself. When you know your worth, it becomes easier to recognize that the rude stares, microaggressions, and negativity you encounter aren't about you—they're about the person throwing them your way.

My greatest joy is seeing that light bulb go off for young people—when they realize that experiencing any kind of "-ism" (like racism, sexism, homophobia, or ableism) is not a reflection of their value. It's a reflection of the person perpetuating those harmful beliefs. That shift in perspective is *revolutionary*, and it can change your life.

Even if you don't have tangible sources of support right now, I want this book to be a constant reminder that *you are enough exactly as you are.* You are here to grow, to learn, and to become a better version of yourself each day—but the paradox is, even as you grow, you are already perfect. The fact that you're still here, persevering in a world that can feel stacked against you, is proof of your strength and brilliance.

Now, while I intended for this book to be for young folks, I definitely won't be mad if it gets the point across to people in other age groups. Believe me, we could all use a good heaping dose of TLC. If you've ever felt like life is a bit too much, or you haven't felt fully heard, or if you're just trying to figure out how to *not completely lose it* when your feelings are all over the map and the world isn't doing a good job of prioritizing your safety, you're in the right place. Heck, as I write this, I'm in my fifties and still working on this stuff! (Yes, even professionals like me are *still* learning how to regulate our emotions, especially when life throws curveballs.)

That's why I've always wished I could teach these skills earlier—so we don't waste our precious energy on self-doubt and confusion when we could be focusing on the things that truly matter to us, no matter how big or small. So no matter your age, if you need to learn how to preserve your mental peace, this book's for you, too.

Rise and Thrive Mindset Remix

In the next several sections, I'll share culturally relevant, grounded, practical tools and compassionate advice to help you quiet the anxiety and self-doubt that might be holding you back.

I mixed this book into seven distinct "mindsets" because they are the secret sauce to living your best life—one that's authentic, empowered, and full of joy. They're not lofty ideals or complicated philosophies—they're down-to-earth tools that anyone can use, no matter where you are on your journey. We're calling them mindsets because they're less like rigid rules and more like a vibrant chemistry set—each one unique, with its own mix of elements you can experiment with. You don't have to use all of them at once; you can "remix" them however you like, creating combinations that suit your moment or mood. These mindsets are about embracing a way of being, like slipping into a well-loved costume that helps you embody a certain energy. They're not instructions to follow but invitations to explore—tools for alchemy, *your own mindset playlist*, both playful and profound, transforming how you move through the world.

I've learned through my own experience that when you name your truth, focus on what matters, create space for yourself, embrace your emotions, turn stress into fuel, and recognize your own worth, everything starts to shift. These mindsets are like the GPS for your soul's journey, guiding you through the ups and downs, helping you grow, and reminding you that you're already everything you need to be. Let's briefly touch on them:

1: Name to Flame, Shame and Blame

Let's get real! Naming our feelings and experiences is like giving shame and blame a one-way ticket out of town. This section shows you how owning your story and embracing your identity can turn the volume down on negativity and set the foundation for lifelong peace and healing. We explore what toxic shame looks like, and how we can move beyond it to claim all parts of our identity.

2: May the Focus Be with You

Ready to channel your inner Jedi? Mastering focus isn't just for monks—it's for everyone who's tired of being distracted. Learn how to laser in on what matters and ditch the mental clutter. In this section, we also cover how to deal with anxiety and ADHD.

3: Hold Space 4 U

You have permission to take up space and center yourself—don't shrink to make others comfortable. In this section, we talk about how depression can cause many of us, especially marginalized young people, to shrink in order to avoid getting hurt—and how we can choose different coping tactics.

4: Ride the Roller Coaster

Life's an emotional amusement park—hold on tight! Learn how to manage the dizzying highs and gut-wrenching lows, and how to stay grounded when you're about to lose your lunch on the emotional loop-de-loop. Here, we talk about conditions involving big feelings (like bipolar disorder and oppositional defiant disorder) and how we can practice emotional regulation.

5: Tend Your Stress, Nurture Your Growth

Stress doesn't have to be your enemy. In fact, it can be your superpower! Discover how to turn the heat up on growth and use stress to fuel your inner superhero. In this section, we cover stress management and how we can also approach phenomena like trauma and grief.

6: You Are a Gift

Guess what? You're a walking, talking, magical gift. This section is all about reminding you of your awesomeness, breaking free from societal pressure, and saying "I'm fabulous" with confidence. Here, we dive into what self-love, self-concept, and self-esteem look like—not just in theory, but in practice.

7: Love Inside, Love Outside

Whether it's with yourself or others, love starts from within. Explore how to create your own love bubble, set boundaries that stick, and build a squad that lifts you up. We'll go over how self-love and love for community can intersect as the strongest support you'll ever have—and you'll be empowered to create it for yourself!

These mindsets aren't just words; they're your keys to living fully, and to make it even easier, each one comes with its own special symbol—think of them as your personal "life emojis." You can use them to quickly remind yourself of each principle, share them with others, or just smile at how simple and fun they are. No fuss, no hassle—just little symbols to guide your way and keep you sparkling!

My hope is that working through all the mindsets will help you see yourself more clearly, understand your unique gifts, and start asking questions about how your mindset shapes your life. We'll explore how to set boundaries (yes, I *see* you trying to please everyone), prioritize your mental health and peace of mind (so you don't end up crying into your pillow every night), and create a stronger sense of solidarity with yourself—all while staying true to who you are.

I want to be real with you: This approach isn't a "paint by numbers" kind of thing. It's not about following a strict, one-size-fits-all formula for feeling better. Mental health is messy, complex, and *so* nonlinear. As you go through this book, you might find yourself experiencing multiple symptoms or challenges at once—maybe one day you're anxious, the next you're feeling isolated, and then a few days later, you're hitting a mental-health high. And guess what? That's totally OK. It's part of the process. What matters is that you're showing up for yourself, and every small step counts. *This is how you remix!*

I also want this to be a resource you can count on and share with your loved ones. Knowledge is power, my friend! And I'm not just talking about knowing the lyrics to every song on TikTok (though that's impressive, too). I'm talking about understanding your mental health and how it affects you—and, yes, the stats and data matter here! Experts and specialists, especially those who look like you and share your experiences, have lots of research and insight to offer. With that knowledge, you can be your own activist, pushing for change in your own life and in your community.

We all have a responsibility to stay well-informed—especially in a world where misinformation is more widespread than that one friend who's always sending you random conspiracy theories. So please get your info from credible sources—and trust me, you're *totally* smart enough to get it. The more you educate yourself, the more you can educate others. You're part of the next generation of mental-health educators, and together, we can spread knowledge and create positive change.

Speaking of change, we're living smack in the middle of some massive shifts, and young people like you are leading the charge. My goal is to equip you for this work by helping you honor your deep inner truth and recognize your immense power. Being seen, heard, and valued is the ultimate way to honor yourself—and guess what? It's *your right*.

This isn't about playing into the toxic hierarchies of "mean girl" or "bro" culture. You don't have to fit into anyone's mold. You have full permission to break the mold, to topple the hierarchies, and to embrace more and more of who you are!

You are part of a beautiful, intricate web of life that has deep and ancient roots, and you deserve to be nourished in every way. Your mental health is a crucial part of your journey to freedom, and I'm here to be your biggest cheerleader. I know the world can feel scary sometimes, and fear has a way of stopping us in our tracks. But I want to help you be brave. I want you to feel the fear and keep moving forward—toward freedom, toward joy, and toward a life that truly reflects who you are.

Please hear me when I tell you, you've got this, and I'm here for it.

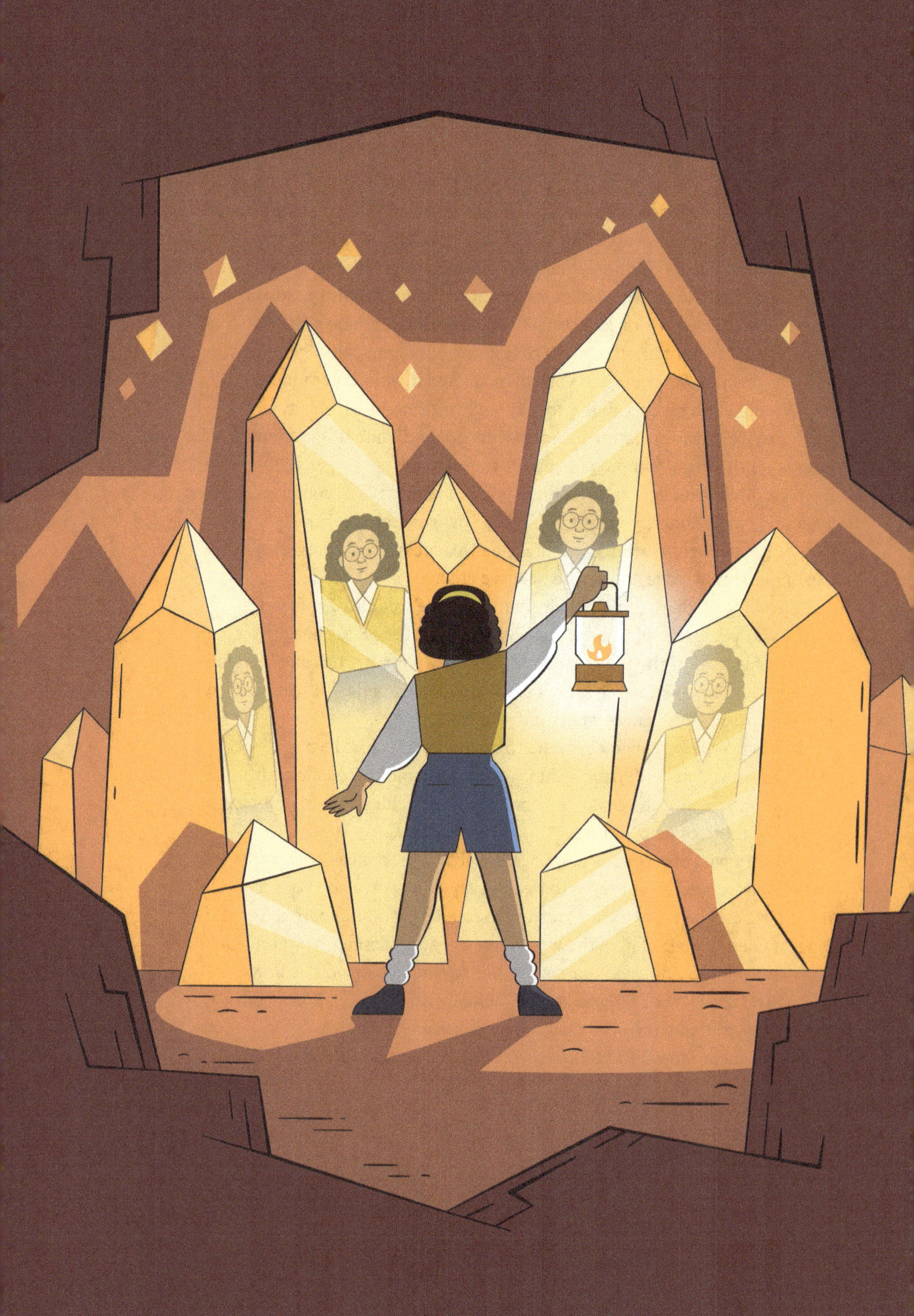

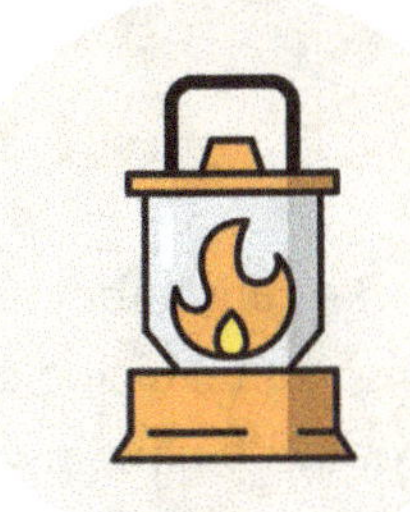

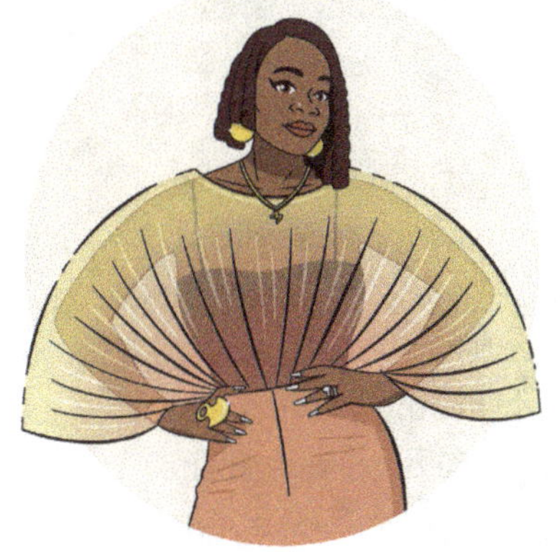

Mindset 1

Name to Flame, Shame and Blame

One of the keys to building your own safe space is naming your thoughts, feelings, emotions, identities, and experiences. This is a powerful act of solidarity with ourselves that has the added benefit of teaching other people how to treat us, as well. Our power rests in our capacity to know that naming what we see in our daily lives, naming what we need to feel safe, naming what feels unsafe for us, etc., gives us information about who we are and what we need. And when we get clear about what we need by taking the time to think about it and name it, we become a safe space for ourselves through our own empowerment. By extension, we show others that we possess the kind of self-awareness to meet any moment of challenge with the tools to adapt and overcome.

By the end of this section, you will know more about:

- Psychological safety (and lack of it)
- Why self-reflection is a beautiful form of self-empowerment
- Why treating yourself as the "standard" is a powerful act of self-love
- The importance of identity—as you choose to define it and in all its complex layers

Let's Get Started

I can remember as far back as junior high how anxious I'd get on Sunday nights. Like clockwork, the feeling crept in every single week. Back then, I couldn't explain why—I just knew it happened. Every. Single. Sunday.

Looking back, though? Oh, I *definitely* know what I was afraid of. I worried about being one of the only two to three Black girls in advanced English, about how my high-school AP history teacher took us to a colonial home and casually told us that Black people could *one day* aspire to live in a place like that. (Yeah, that actually happened.) I worried about how my tenth-grade crush—who all my friends had *strategically* arranged for me to sit next to on the bus after a football game—literally pushed me out of the seat. (Also a true story. And yes, it was brutal and awful.) I worried about navigating friend groups made up of different races, always trying to find my place, to belong. And on and on it went.

I didn't *have* a name for those feelings until I was well into adulthood. All I knew was that Sunday nights felt eerie, unsettling. That unease followed me well into my thirties.

Then, one day, I learned the term *Sunday Scaries.* This refers to that antsy, uneasy feeling that creeps in on Sunday nights when you start stressing about the week ahead. It's like a mini dread-fest—your brain suddenly remembers all the homework, work deadlines, awkward social situations, or responsibilities waiting for you on Monday. Even if you had a great weekend, the Sunday Scaries can sneak up, making you feel restless, nervous, or overwhelmed.

And just like that, I wasn't alone. I wasn't weird or broken for feeling this way. I wasn't the only person who dreaded Sundays, who felt their stomach tighten at the thought of the week ahead. And once I could *name* my fears, I could face them. I stopped blaming myself. I let go of the shame. And I realized—I was going to be OK.

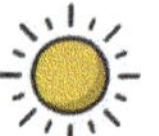 ## What Is Psychological Safety?

Safety can be defined as the condition of feeling protected from harm or risk. While it is ideal for us all to experience safety, for a lot of young people, it can feel hard to come by. Safety is an important building block for our mental health—we need to feel safe and free from judgment, punishment, or retaliation in order to freely express ourselves, our feelings, and our wishes and desires. As my story demonstrates, one way we create safety for ourselves is by naming things that once lurked in the dark—giving words to our fears, anxieties, and unspoken experiences. When we name something, we shine a light on it, making it feel more manageable and less overwhelming. This is how we create safety for ourselves.

Psychological safety is something we feel on the inside when we experience external spaces (home, school, an after-school program) that are consciously designed to make us feel safe. Safe spaces allow us to be our bravest selves, so we should recognize that while external safe spaces are not always possible, this book will help you explore the power of building your own psychologically safe and supportive community (even if that community is just you and one other person).

I want to dig in deeper and give you two specific models for psychological safety: internal and external. Think of **internal safety** as what *you* can control—it's about how you treat yourself, how you talk to yourself, and how much you trust yourself. It includes things like self-acceptance, confidence, and knowing that your body and mind belong to *you*. Basically, it's about creating a safe space *within yourself*.

External safety, on the other hand, is about what's happening around you—the things other people control or influence. This includes how safe you feel at school, in your friend group, at home, or on social media. Some parts of external safety you can shape, and some you can't.

Here's the important part: Even when you *can't* control everything around you (like whether your family fully accepts you or you're being bullied or trolled by a classmate), you *can* control how you take care of yourself internally.

For example, let's say lunchtime at school feels unsafe because there's one kid who always has something nasty to say to you. You might love hanging out with the rest of the group, but that one person makes it exhausting. You have the power to decide: *Do I keep sitting there? Do I find another place to eat?* You can't force that kid to be kind, but you *can* choose how much space you give them in your life.

Building internal safety means treating yourself the way you'd treat your best friend. You wouldn't let someone talk down to them, right? So why let yourself absorb that kind of negativity? You'd remind them they're too amazing to waste energy on people who can't be consistently kind—and you deserve that reminder, too.

At the end of the day, you always have an *internal* point of control (which basically means you can decide how much power something has over you). Even when everything around you feels shaky, you can always turn inward and find small moments of safety. And sometimes, those small moments—deep breaths, a song that comforts you, a reassuring thought—are enough to carry you through the hardest days.

You don't have to control everything to protect your peace. You just have to hold on to what's *yours*.

🏮 JOURNAL PROMPT

How do you think naming difficult emotions or experiences might help to create a sense of psychological safety?

Signs of Psychological Unsafety

Psychological unsafety isn't just about someone being openly mean or hurtful—it's when you don't feel comfortable being yourself because you're afraid of being judged, embarrassed, or shut down. It's also not just about obvious negativity; it's also when people ignore, dismiss, or discourage you, making it hard to speak up, take risks, or feel like you truly belong. Below are some signs that you are feeling and experiencing psychological unsafety:

 **Fear of speaking up:** You worry that sharing your thoughts or feelings will lead to judgment, embarrassment, or negative consequences.

 **Feeling ignored or dismissed:** Your ideas, concerns, or emotions are brushed off, making you feel like your voice doesn't matter.

 **Constant self-censorship:** You hold back from expressing yourself because you're afraid of how others will react.

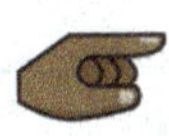 **Blame and shame culture:** Mistakes aren't treated as learning experiences but as things to be punished or ridiculed for.

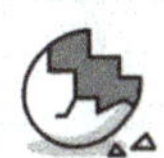 **Walking on eggshells:** You feel like you always have to be extra careful with what you say or do to avoid conflict or criticism.

 **Exclusion or isolation:** You feel left out, unwelcome, or like you don't truly belong in the space you're in.

 **High stress and anxiety:** Just being in the environment makes you tense, anxious, or mentally drained.

Signs of Psychological Safety

Feeling truly safe isn't just about the absence of harm or discomfort—it's about the active creation of a space where you <u>know</u> you're supported and can be yourself. It's not just about what's <u>not</u> happening (like judgment or negativity); it's about the things that <u>are</u> happening—like kindness, respect, and trust—so you feel secure speaking up, making mistakes, and being yourself. Below are some signs that you are feeling and experiencing psychological safety:

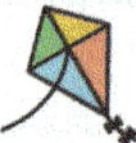 **A sense of ease:** You feel calm, knowing you won't be judged or punished for expressing yourself

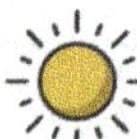 **A clear mind:** You can think and make decisions without fear clouding your judgment

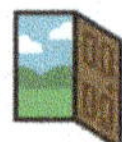 **An open door:** You feel comfortable sharing your thoughts, ideas, and emotions without hesitation

 **Courage to take risks:** You're not afraid to try new things, even if there's a chance of failure

 **Confidence to speak up:** You feel secure voicing your opinions because you know your voice matters

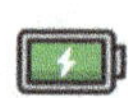 **Drive to take action:** You feel inspired to participate, contribute, and make things happen without fear holding you back

 **A sense of belonging:** You feel welcomed, and you're fully present, interested, and connected to what's happening around you

Here's a QR code that'll take you to two different videos that help you create a sense of psychological safety so you can be yourself, take risks, and thrive!

🏮 JOURNAL PROMPT

Can you recall a time when you felt truly safe and secure, both internally and externally? Take a moment to write it down. Think about where you were, who you were with, what you were doing, and how this sense of safety felt in your mind and body. How did you respond to it? If you can write down answers to all these questions, you can better understand what psychological safety feels like—and how it can support your well-being and resilience. (Extra credit for creating a list of specific things you can do to make yourself feel psychologically safe!)

Sunshine Is the Best Disinfectant

Sunshine is the best disinfectant. My brother told me that once, and I've never forgotten it. When we shine a light on something, we can see it clearly. And when we see it clearly, we can understand it. Naming things— especially parts of ourselves that have been pushed into the shadows—is one of the most important things you can do to create safety. It's a way of saying, "I see you. I honor you." That's why naming our identities matters. We need to see them, understand them, and then, most importantly, embrace and love every single part of who we are.

Our identities shape how we see the world and how the world sees us. Race, gender, sexuality, ability, immigration status—even something as simple as having a name that people refuse to learn—can all affect our experiences. Some identities are treated as the "default," while others are marginalized. But that doesn't mean we should shrink ourselves to fit in. Instead, we need to call it what it is and push back against it. We need to stand firm in who we are.

You are not marginal—you have been marginalized. And there's a big difference.

One way I personally resist this is by capitalizing the phrase **People of Color**. It's my way of saying we are not small. We are the **global majority**—powerful, unshakable, and unwilling to be diminished.

There's a word for the way our different identities overlap and shape our experiences: **intersectionality**. Professor Kimberlé Crenshaw created the term to help us remember that none of us is just *one* thing. We are layered. We are multifaceted. If you hold even one marginalized identity, your experiences will be different from someone who holds none. And while no two people's lives are exactly the same, there are struggles that many of us share—like having our names constantly mispronounced, being asked where we're *really* from, having our accomplishments dismissed as "handouts," or being denied the right to identify as we truly are. When you carry multiple marginalized identities, the fight for psychological safety grows even harder.

So how do you push back? How do you create safety when the world tells you that parts of who you are don't belong?

You name yourself. You claim yourself. You step into your truth.

When you fully embrace who you are, you create internal safety. You stop blaming and shaming yourself. You make peace with your reflection. You light a spark of clarity that no one can take from you. Think of a trans teen finally stepping into their identity, even when others refuse to see them for who they are. That's an act of self-affirmation, of choosing to stand in their truth, no matter what the world says. That's what naming yourself can do.

But finding psychological safety outside of yourself takes strategy. You have to look at your surroundings and ask: *Who can I trust? Who sees me? What tools do I need to feel safe? Where are my allies? Who has been through this before and can help me navigate it?*

Naming ourselves, our beauty, and our worth is an act of defiance. It's a reminder that who you are is not just OK—it is powerful. But let's be real—society, and sometimes even family, feeds us messages that tell us otherwise. And when you've heard those messages your whole life, they become your guardrails, shaping how you see yourself. That's why we have to challenge them, unlearn them, and replace them with something new.

The truth is, being strong in your identity can sometimes create distance between you and others. And while you should never accept abuse or erasure, there may be moments when finding common ground is necessary. If you can hold onto your identity and still maintain a relationship, then it's worth figuring out how.

At the end of the day, naming yourself is an act of power. It's an act of love. And when you do it, you make space for others to do the same.

The Mosaic of Identity

Identity tells us who we are. It's shaped over time, influenced by both internal and external factors, and constantly evolving. Sometimes we feel

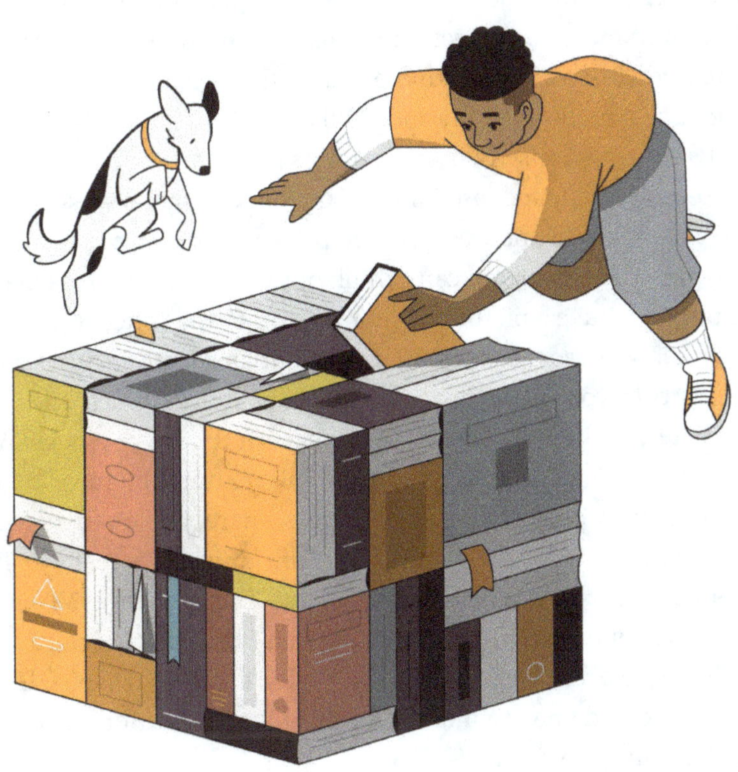

The mosaic of identity

like we know ourselves completely, and other times, parts of us feel like a mystery. But at our core, there's always something steady—something that stays *us*, even as everything else shifts.

We're going to dig deep into identity—what it means, how it forms, and why it matters. To start, think about all the identities that shape you: race, ethnicity, gender identity, sexual orientation, age, ability, socioeconomic status, religion, language, immigration status, and more. These pieces make up the unique mosaic of *you*.

One powerful way to understand identity is by creating an *identity mosaic*—a way to visualize and claim all the parts that make us who we are. Too often, young people are boxed in by expectations: *Boys do this, girls do that. Latinos act one way, Asians another.* Sometimes, people refuse to acknowledge certain identities at all, trying to erase them. But here's the truth: Your identity is yours to define. No one else gets to tell you who you are.

Think of the identity mosaic like a 3D puzzle. Each piece represents a core part of *you*. When all the pieces are together, they create a complete picture. But if a piece is missing, stolen, or hidden, there's a hole where it should be. And sometimes, to feel safe, we *do* hide pieces—maybe to avoid conflict, to fit in, or to protect ourselves from harm. But my hope is that you can find (or create) the kind of safety that allows you to show up *fully* as yourself—unapologetically and brilliantly.

Let's try an exercise right now, in this moment.

Take a piece of paper and draw a large blocky shape—like a puzzle with twelve pieces. Write one word in each piece that represents an important part of your identity. If you can't think of twelve, start with as many as come to mind. Take a picture of your first draft and reflect on it for a few minutes. Now, erase the words. Think about an *average* day in your life. Which parts of your identity do you show the most? Which ones do you keep quieter? Write the identities you share in the *larger* blocks. Write the ones you hide in the *smaller* blocks. Take another picture. Look at the differences. Why do some parts feel safe to share, while others feel risky?

This exercise helps us see just how *complex* identity really is. It shifts in different situations, and that's OK. But what never changes? There is only one you. Out of *billions* of people, no one else has your exact mix of identities. If we gave every person in the world the same twelve puzzle pieces to arrange, we'd end up with more than six quintillion different combinations. That's how unique you are.

Now that you've mapped out your identity, let's talk about something that can hold us back: *shame.*

When we're constantly fighting to be seen—fighting to exist in spaces that try to erase us—it can take a toll. It can lead to anxiety, depression, and self-doubt. We might start questioning if we're too much, not enough, or somehow "wrong." And if we don't check those thoughts, they can turn into deep shame.

Sometimes, shame comes from the world around us. Imagine being an immigrant with an accent and hearing people mock the way you speak. Or being compared to someone who struggles *a little* but doesn't face the same discrimination as you. These experiences pile up, making us question ourselves.

And then there's *comparison*. Social media makes it worse—we see perfect lives, perfect bodies, perfect relationships. But here's the truth: The only person you are the standard for is YOU. Your only job is to be the best version of *yourself*, not someone else.

Speaking of being you: Ever noticed how you speak one way with your friends, another way with teachers, and maybe another with family? That's *code-switching*—something we all do. But for marginalized folks, it's more than just changing tones. It can be the difference between feeling safe and feeling exposed.

Imagine a gay teen walking into a barbershop, unsure if it's queer-friendly. He might present himself as more traditionally "masculine" until he knows it's safe to be himself. But the moment he sees another LGBTQAI+ person in the shop, he might relax. That's code-switching for safety.

Recognizing these shifts is important. It helps us understand why we sometimes hide parts of ourselves—and reminds us that *our full selves* deserve to be seen.

Just remember: You are a mosaic—a living, breathing work of art, filled with beautiful and complex pieces. Whether you're bicultural, multilingual, first-generation, or anything else, those pieces make you *one in eight billion*. You were never meant to fit into someone else's mold because *you are the mold*.

So take everything in this section, let it fuel you, and step into the world knowing that your identity is *yours* to own, celebrate, and protect.

Now, let's keep going. We've got more to explore.

🏮 JOURNAL PROMPT

What are some aspects of your identity that feel important to you? Write them down, even if they're things you've never shared with anyone. How does it feel to name these parts of yourself? Does it feel empowering, scary, or something else? Why do you think that is?

Think about the different parts of your identity, like your culture, race, gender, abilities, or the way you express yourself. Which parts have shaped your life the most? Have you ever felt like one of these parts of your identity made things easier or harder for you? Describe a time this happened.

Have you ever felt like someone didn't understand your experiences because they didn't share your identity? What did that feel like? Think about a time when you met someone with a different identity than yours. What did you learn from them? How were your experiences similar, and how were they different?

Why do you think it's important to give yourself permission to name your identities? Write about a time when you spoke up about an important part of who you are. What happened? How did it make you feel? If you could tell the world one thing about yourself that you think they need to know, what would it be?

Normalizing You

As we've already talked about (and as it bears repeating), the only person you are the standard for is *you*. Getting behind yourself means fully owning your identity—not just the parts that others accept or expect, but all of it. Too often, we're taught that we have to fit into some kind of mold, as if there's one "right" way to be. But that's a lie. There *is no mold*. You are not here to squeeze yourself into someone else's idea of who you should be. You are here to be *you*.

But here's where it gets tricky—shame is constantly hiding out, sometimes in places we don't expect, and like a nasty jack-in-the-box, it can pop up . . . sometimes, right when we think we've got it all figured out. Shame, especially toxic shame, doesn't just make us feel bad—it can rewire the way we see ourselves.

Unlike regular shame, which might come and go when we make a mistake, toxic shame *sticks*. It's the difference between *I did something wrong* and *there's something wrong with me*. It convinces us that we are unworthy, unlovable, or broken at our core. Instead of helping us grow or change, it traps us in self-doubt, self-blame, and a constant feeling of not being enough. Toxic shame isn't just an emotion—it's a weight that follows us, shaping our thoughts, our choices, and even the way we move through the world.

It can make us believe we're fundamentally broken, instead of understanding that we are just *different,* not defective. And when we internalize that message, it doesn't just sit there quietly. We start fighting ourselves.

That fight is exhausting. And it has real consequences. When you're constantly at war with yourself—telling yourself you should be *less this, more that, different somehow*—it takes a toll. That kind of internal conflict contributes to anxiety and depression. Sometimes, a specific event (bullying, discrimination, rejection) can push you into full-on self-blame and shame. And in some cases, repeated experiences of rejection or oppression can lead to PTSD. This is why understanding how we process our emotions, and how we hold space for *ourselves,* is so important.

Psychology gives us a way to look at this: adaptive vs. maladaptive responses. Adaptive responses are the healthy ones that help us move through challenges. Maladaptive responses are the ones that keep us stuck, making things harder instead of easier. But something to keep in mind here is that what's considered "maladaptive" is often judged by a dominant culture that doesn't account for different ways of being.

White supremacy, for example, tells you that you should be "normal"—but whose definition of normal are we talking about? Many of us come from cultures with their own ways of being, their own ways of thinking, healing, and processing the world. Just because something is seen as "disordered" in one culture doesn't mean it's actually wrong. That's why I don't want us to fixate on rigid categories of mental-health "disorders" as if they are absolute. Instead, we ask: *What is working? What actually helps?*

This is why we have to be careful about how we label ourselves. It's not about rejecting diagnoses or ignoring symptoms—it's about calibrating to what *serves us.* If you have OCD, ADHD, or anything else, the goal isn't to erase those parts of you or force yourself into a "normal" that wasn't designed with you in mind. The goal is to understand what *you* need and how *you* function best. Labels can be useful tools, but they should never become cages.

So let's reframe it. You are not a problem to be fixed. You are not broken. Your job isn't to mold yourself into what the world wants—it's to figure out what allows *you* to thrive. The only standard you need to meet is your own.

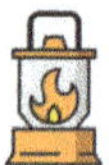 # JOURNAL PROMPT

Think about a time when you felt like you had to act, look, or be a certain way just to fit in. What was that like? Who or what made you feel that way?

Now, say this to yourself: "The only person I am the standard for is me." What does that mean to you? How would you feel if you didn't have to follow anyone else's idea of who you should be?

Picture a version of you that's 100 percent unapologetically YOU—no pretending, no shame, just owning every part of who you are. What does that person look like? Do they look like you? How does it feel to imagine being that person? What is one thing you can do today to help you step into that version of yourself?

Toxic Blame & Shame in Marginalized Young People

We've talked a lot about getting behind ourselves—fully owning who we are—and how shame can get in the way of that. But shame doesn't exist in a vacuum. Toxic shame and self-blame are often tied to experiences like racial trauma, discrimination, and the constant pressure to conform to standards that were never made for us. When the world repeatedly sends messages that who you are is *wrong* or *less than*, it doesn't just hurt in the moment—it can shape the way you see yourself in the long term. That's why I want to take a moment to share some research that makes it clear just how real these struggles are.

Through my nonprofit, we conduct a periodic study called *The State of Mental Health of Youth and Young Adults of Color* (SOMHYC).[1] In 2025, we ran the second version of this study, and what we found about stereotypes and coping among Youth of Color was eye-opening. Let's be clear: *stereotypes affect everyone*, but they don't affect everyone in the same way. Some people can brush them off, while for others, they have real, lasting consequences—especially for marginalized young people.

---

1. Breland-Noble, A., The AAKOMA Project, and C. A. Harb. *State of Mental Health of Youth and Young Adults of Color, Full Report*. 2025.

AAKOMA's research showed that:

- **8.7%** of youth reported experiencing racial trauma *often or very often* in the past year from teachers or employers.
- **11.3%** of all youth reported experiencing racial trauma *often or very often* from peers or friends.
- **25.8%** of Youth of Color reported experiencing racial trauma *often or very often* from social media.[2]

We also found that:

- **40.4%** of youth had people say negative things about their race.
- **17.1%** of youth were bullied online about their sexual orientation.
- **20.9%** of youth had mean or rude comments posted about their weight.[3]

Now, imagine being bombarded with messages like this all the time. When that happens over and over, it can seep in, becoming a part of how you see yourself. That's *toxic shame*. And the worst part? It usually targets things we *can't* and *shouldn't* change about ourselves.

This is why our identity mosaic is so important. It helps protect us against these attacks by reminding us of the things that make us *powerful*. When people try to tear us down, we need something to ground us—something that reminds us of our worth. That's where our superpowers come in. Our multilayered, brilliant, and unique identity is our greatest defense.

So the next time toxic shame shows up, ask yourself: *Which of my superpowers will I use to defeat it?*

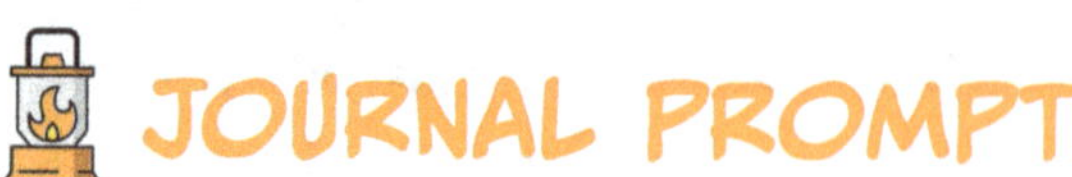

JOURNAL PROMPT

Shame often tries to convince us that we don't belong or that we're "too much" or "not enough." What's one lie shame has told you about your identity? What's the truth you know in your heart, even if it feels hard to believe sometimes?

---

2. Breland-Noble, A., The AAKOMA Project, and C. A. Harb. *State of Mental Health of Youth and Young Adults of Color, Full Report.* 2025.

3. Breland-Noble, A., The AAKOMA Project, and C. A. Harb. *State of Mental Health of Youth and Young Adults of Color, Full Report.* 2025.

Finally, think about how the unique parts of your identity are a source of strength, resilience, and beauty. What are your special superpowers that nobody else but you has?

I Don't Feel Safe—How Do I Help Myself?

It's hard to open up, to relax, or to feel like you belong when you don't feel emotionally safe. You might keep your guard up, not because you want to—but because life has taught you that being real or vulnerable isn't always safe. Maybe you've been ignored, judged, or shut down when you tried to share what's real for you. Maybe you've been told that your feelings are "too much."

You already know how exhausting it is to keep yourself on lockdown all the time. But for a lot of us, it starts to feel normal. Like the only way to survive is to shrink, numb out, or act like everything's fine when it's not. But I'm here to remind you that your truth is your power. It's like your internal compass. But if you don't feel safe, it's hard to trust that compass—or even hear it.

The first step is to check in with where you're really at. That might sound basic, but emotional safety isn't something you can force. You can't fake it. You have to *sense* it. It's kind of like walking into a room and instantly feeling whether you're welcome. You can feel it in your body, even if no one says anything out loud.

So ask yourself: *Am I OK with always hiding what I feel or who I am just to keep the peace?*

If you're reading this, chances are your answer is "no."

Now, ask yourself the next question: *Am I ready to do one thing to feel a little more emotionally safe?* That might mean being more honest—with yourself first. It might mean naming what you need, or finding one person who sees you clearly.

If your answer is "not yet," that's OK, too. Sometimes, you've had to survive by staying quiet. Sometimes, your nervous system is on high alert all the time. Sometimes, the people around you have made it unsafe to be your full self. And if you hold a marginalized identity, that layer of emotional unsafety can feel even deeper. Maybe the world sees you through stereotypes. Maybe your family or community hasn't made space for who you are. Maybe you've never heard someone say that your feelings matter. But they do. You matter. And emotional safety isn't just for other people—it's for you, too.

Let's talk about ways to start creating it—slowly, on your terms.

1. **Start by being honest—with *yourself*.** You don't have to share everything with others right away. But in your own mind, in your journal, or in quiet moments, tell the truth about how you feel. That truth is sacred. It's where healing begins.

2. **Notice who feels safe—and who doesn't.** Who listens when you speak? Who makes space for your emotions, instead of shutting them down? You don't need a crowd. Even one person who honors your truth can change everything. You might find acceptance in an online community, a group at school, a creative space, or a friend's living room. Look for places where you don't have to edit yourself to fit in. These are your oxygen zones.

3. **Let your body be part of the conversation.** Emotional safety isn't just about your thoughts—it lives in your body. Notice when you tense up, when you freeze, or when you feel that little bit of ease. Your body often knows before your brain does.

4. **Create rituals that help you feel grounded.** Light a candle. Listen to music that understands you. Write a list of things you *won't* apologize for. Make a playlist of songs that feel like emotional armor. These small practices help you claim your space—inside and out.

5. **Self-reflect.** Forget what other people tell you to like or dislike. What actually brings you joy? What are your natural strengths? What motivates you? What makes you feel safe? What drains you? Understanding these things about yourself will help you figure out what coping strategies will actually work for you.

JOURNAL PROMPT

Which of the suggestions for helping yourself lit you up the most? Why? In what ways can you start incorporating them into your life to be more aligned with your whole identity and your true self?

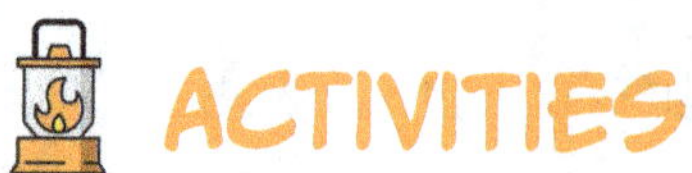

ACTIVITIES

Now that you know something about psychological safety and ways to embrace your unique identity, let's practice some new skills.

EASY

Name Your Identities

Take a moment to name every identity that you hold. And I mean *all* of them: the small ones, the big ones, and everything in between. Then rank them in order, based on most significant with respect to how they've shown up in your life this week (i.e., at the forefront of your mind every single day) to least significant (i.e., you didn't even think about it).

After this activity, I feel:

MODERATE

Representations of You

Find a movie, TV show, podcast, etc., with a character or person who shares one of the most important aspects of your identity (e.g., an LGBTQAI+ character or a podcast with a host that speaks to these issues regularly). Watch the movie/listen to the podcast, then spend one week in reflection for five minutes a day, just thinking about how the images you've seen and the things you've heard impact you emotionally. Do you feel seen when you watch this person? Do you feel the depiction/presentation is accurate? What do you wish was different to make the character/person more reflective of your own lived experience with this shared identity?

After this activity, I feel:

HARD

Contemplating What You've Been Taught

Ask a loved one you trust to talk with you about their philosophy on teaching you about your racial, ethnic, gender, etc., identity when you were a child. This is an adult who values the person you are (the exercise works best when you know they accept and love you unconditionally). If you can't find that person and this exercise isn't something that's safe for you right now, it's totally fine to skip it.

If you have that adult in your life, ask them why they taught you certain things and not others (for example, many kids of immigrant families may have parents/caregivers who do not teach the children their language of origin as a means of helping children assimilate). Once you hear your loved one's story about why they taught you certain things about your identity and left out others, journal about it. Identify your emotional and sensational states as you listened to them share their story. What was the impact on you in the moment? How has the messaging they taught you played out in your life? How has it impacted other parts of your identity, for better or worse?

After this activity, I feel:

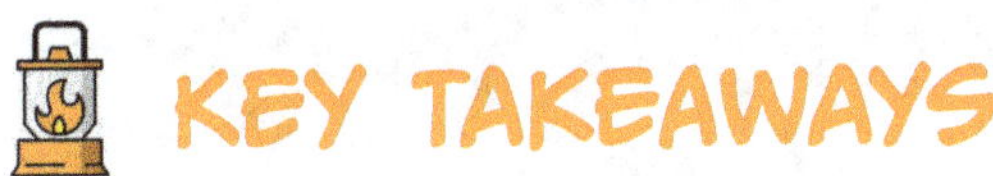 # KEY TAKEAWAYS

Congrats! You made it to the end of Mindset 1: Name to Flame, Shame and Blame! Have you learned anything you want to incorporate into your daily routine? Is there anything in this section you want to shout from the rooftops about? Maybe you've learned something you can share with your friends or parents/caregivers to help them. Make a note of your key takeaways (including the ones you'd like to share with others) and write them below:

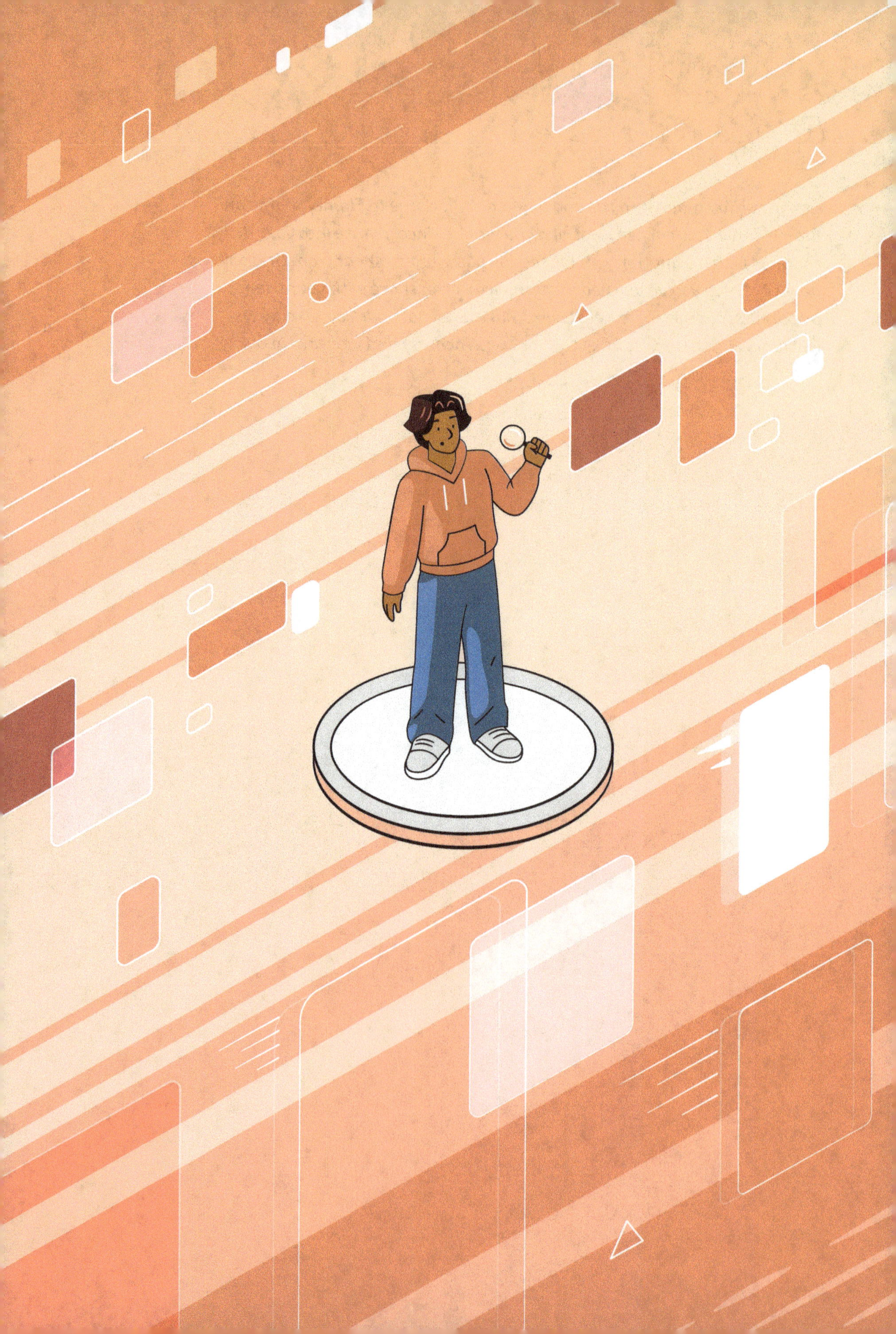

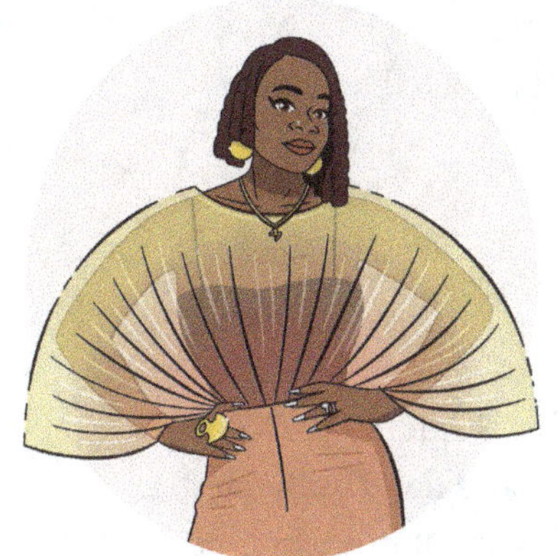

Mindset 2

May the Focus Be with You

Everyone is dealing with distractions or feelings that can leave us unfocused. Naturally, it's hard to concentrate on what matters to us if we're busy worrying about the future or analyzing the past. Give yourself grace (i.e., patient, loving kindness) and know that you can lighten your load by switching up what you're focusing on. Focus is not always easy when there are a million little things clamoring for attention, but the million little things should never be in a position to call the shots when it comes to your mental health.

Even when the weight of worry and distraction feels heavy, you can practice "strength training" for your mind and emotions by changing where you place your attention. You don't have to make more space for worries to gain outsized importance in your day to day. Instead, you can start and end the day by focusing your thoughts and emotions in the places that support you. In this section, you'll learn how to use the focus to blast away the stuff that sucks you in and makes you go: *Wait, what happened? Where did all my time and energy go?*

By the end of this section, you will know more about:

- Anxiety, what it is, and how to reduce/prevent it
- Why it's so important to normalize anxiety for everyone, especially for people with marginalized identities
- Active coping skills for empowering yourself to take back your focus, be present, and find your center

Let's Get Started

Maven is a high-school sophomore and one of the few Students of Color at her school. Despite being friendly and sweet, she faces daily bullying from a group of girls in her English class. The bullying escalates when one girl puts her feet on Maven's chair for two days straight. Frustrated and angry, Maven confides in her mom, asking for help. Her mom suggests that Maven advocate for herself first. Together, they devise a plan to address the situation.

They discuss Maven's feelings about the bullying and the lack of support from classmates. They practice what she will say to stand up for herself and reinforce the importance of communicating her needs. After some deep breathing, they focus on Maven's primary goals: stopping the bullying and reducing anxiety. The next day, Maven bravely confronts the group of girls, saying, "Move your feet out of my seat now, and do not let this happen again because I don't like it." The girls comply, and from then on, Maven experiences no further issues with them for the rest of the school year.

Maven did three key things to help herself: she named her trauma and anxiety, she asked for help, and she focused on active coping. Doing all of this empowered Maven to advocate for herself, not only to resolve her immediate problem but also to show her ability to face her anxiety with focus and a plan.

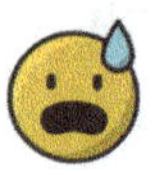 What Is Anxiety?

We hear lots of people talk about anxiety, describing it as knots or butterflies in their stomach, sweaty palms, or a rapid heartbeat. If you've ever felt this way, I want you to know that *everyone* experiences anxiety because it is a perfectly ordinary response to an unpredictable world. Anxiety is an uncomfortable feeling of fear or imminent disaster—and a normal emotional response to danger. The American Psychological Association describes anxiety as "emotions characterized by feelings of tension, worried thoughts, and even physical changes like increased blood pressure."[4]

While we all know what anxiety feels like, we do not all experience it with the same intensity. And it's when our anxiety causes problems like changing our eating and sleeping habits, making us feel irritable, or making it hard for us to concentrate that we need to take charge and acknowledge it more deeply.

Anxiety is born out of our natural fight-or-flight response, which is our body's reaction to a perceived threat. But a mind that gets stuck in fight-or-flight is the type that we label as anxious. Anxious thoughts can be conscious, or they can buzz around in our subconscious, like a soundtrack on repeat (even if it's at a super-low volume). When our fight-or-flight response goes into overdrive, it can become **maladaptive** (the opposite of helpful). At that point, anxiety drifts into the realm of a disorder and becomes something in need of loving care. Sometimes, our behaviors help—other times, they reinforce anxiety. However, we can reduce flare-ups as soon as they start.

I want to pause here and ensure that you understand how anxiety and anxiety disorders can show up in our daily lives. Just know that if you're feeling anxious right now, you're not alone—and you deserve support to help you manage.

Here is a QR code to a video where I briefly go over these topics.

---

4. American Psychological Association, "Definition of Anxiety," American Psychological Association, n.d., https://www.apa.org/topics/anxiety.

🔍 JOURNAL PROMPT

Can you recall a time when you felt really worried? Take a moment and write it down. Think about where you were, who you were with, what you were doing, and how the worry felt in your mind and body. How did you respond to it? If you can write down answers to all these questions, you know what it feels like to experience anxiety—and to cope with it in the best ways you knew how at the time.

Signs and Symptoms of Anxiety

Anxiety can sneak up on us in all kinds of ways—sometimes loud and obvious, sometimes quiet and sneaky. Everyone experiences it differently, so take a moment to think about how it shows up for you and add your own to the list below.

Here are some common signs that anxiety might be making itself at home in your body and mind:

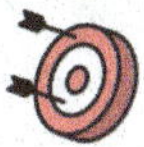 Trouble concentrating or staying present

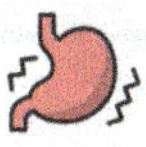 Stomach aches or digestive issues that seem to come out of nowhere

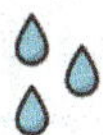 Excessive sweating (even when you're not hot)

 Muscle tension—like your whole body is bracing for something

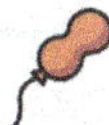 Shallow breathing or feeling like you can't get enough air

 Feeling restless, like you need to be doing something

 Trouble making decisions, even small ones

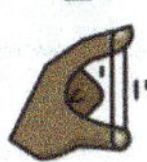 Feeling tense, like you're on edge but don't know why

 Feeling like the world is either speeding up or slowing way down

 Thoughts looping on repeat, no matter how hard you try to stop them

 Obsessing over the past or future instead of focusing on right now

 Constantly worrying that something bad is about to happen

 Playing out worst-case scenarios in your head (and believing them)

Add yours below:

🔍 JOURNAL PROMPT

Have you ever felt anxious, to the point that you experienced any of the signs above? What were the situations or circumstances that brought on those thoughts, emotions, and sensations? Remember, anxiety can be brought on by any number of things—from a math test you didn't have time to study for, to a troubling situation with a friend or family member, to intense worry after reading a story about a school shooting or another Black or Brown child being shot by the people in society who are supposed to protect them. Be gentle with yourself. Everyone reacts to these situations in their own individual ways, but anxiety is a perfectly normal response to life's unpredictability.

Normalizing Anxiety

Have you ever talked to someone who was obviously not OK, but when you asked about how they were *really* doing, they just looked at you and insisted, "I'm fine"? The "I'm fine" response is often a coping behavior that can make us feel like we're in control of a bad situation even when we do not feel in control, so we must be careful with how we speak about our experiences.

Remember what you learned in the first section of this book? The way to beat blaming and shaming is *naming*! That is, when you make time to be 100 percent honest about who you are, where you are, and what you're feeling, you can get behind yourself and seek the support you need. You have it within you to be courageous and pay attention to what's really happening inside you. When you do this, you are better able to fight the automatic response, "I'm fine," when life is everything but.

Sometimes, people think they're hardwired to always be on edge and that there's nothing they can do about it. This is simply not the case because there are many things you *can* do to help yourself. You can learn skills to help you recognize and reduce anxiety and free yourself from its fog and crushing weight—I promise!

🔍 JOURNAL PROMPT

If you find yourself spinning in the lather-rinse-repeat cycle of uncontrolled anxiety, maybe you can think of a time when you felt peace and ease—you were present and focused on what was happening in the moment. What was going on? In thinking about it, how does that change your thoughts, emotions, and feelings right now?

Anxiety in Marginalized Young People

There's an elephant in the room we need to talk about, and it's the fact that we know too little about how anxiety and anxiety disorders look in diverse young people.

People of Color, including those with multiple marginalized identities (LGBTQAI+ , disabled, under-resourced, immigrants, etc.) experience excessive worry about their own safety, the safety of people in their communities, and the safety of their families. For too many marginalized people, safety isn't an abstract thought about the past or future—it's a daily concern.

While everyone experiences challenges that might contribute to anxiety, there are degrees to which marginalized people experience unique stressors that others don't. On top of that, those with intersectional identities (e.g., a low-income young trans Person of Color with invisible disabilities) are often exposed to the added effect of stress related to multiple aspects of their identity. For example, the killings of POC and/ or LGBTQAI+ people—sometimes targeted, sometimes random, almost always unreasonable—and their repeated sharing via social media can make it difficult for members of these communities to feel safe. Repeated exposure to identity-based trauma can have severely damaging effects on a person's anxiety.

We rarely discuss these deeper truths about anxiety and anxiety disorders. Sometimes, we are unaware of them. But these experiences, feelings, and behaviors are very real. And we set ourselves up for successful coping when we're open to learning about emotional well-being and mental health in our communities—and when we gain new strategies that we can regularly, actively practice.

 ## JOURNAL PROMPT

Are there ways your own identities—and, more importantly, the way others have treated you because of how they perceived your identities—have led to feelings of worry, anxiety, or lack of safety? Write down all your feelings— naming them empowers you to take action to uplift yourself and others going through the same experiences.

I Have Anxiety—How Do I Help Myself?

It's hard to "smell the roses" and focus on one thing at a time when your mind is in overdrive and your body's feeling it, too. I like to say that your attention is your currency—and yes, maybe even more important than money! The first step requires that you think about how ready you are to make a change. I know that sounds strange, but you can't make lasting change if you don't have a clue as to whether you're ready. If you wanted to try out for a sport you never played before, you'd have to get yourself ready, right? You'd need to understand the basic rules and probably observe people who are good at playing the sport. In other words, information without motivation is not very useful.

You can estimate your readiness by asking yourself: *Am I OK with my attention and focus going to my anxiety, worry, or (fill in the blank with whatever feels right here)?*

I'm guessing that if you're reading this book, the answer is no!

But then, you have to answer the next question: *Am I ready to do something to shift my attention and focus?*

If your answer is no, maybe you have a little more work to do before taking back your most valuable currency. Sometimes, we say no out of fear; other times, it's because we feel we're too busy; and at others, because we don't want to feel so alone in our struggle. Sometimes, it's because the people around us are discouraging. In addition, if we have marginalized identities, we may have never heard people discuss anxiety, much less how to manage it. We worry that sharing our concerns about the "mental spin" may be met with lack of understanding.

This makes sense. For example, in many Families of Color, we're far less likely to have conversations about mental-health supports. We might encounter family members who don't get it, but we have a duty to care for ourselves, anyway. Poor emotional well-being and mental illness are nothing to be ashamed of, nor should we let stigma prevent us from taking care of ourselves or seeking help. Instead, we (yes, even young people) can be pioneers in our families and communities by making the brave choice to acknowledge our condition and seek support.

Let's discuss some methods to help you take back your focus.

1. **Be present.** This is about being still and allowing your thoughts to flow freely. Mindfulness, meditation, and breathwork are some of the ways we find presence. Journaling can also be a powerful way to quiet the "monkey mind" (racing thoughts of worry and stress). Being present helps you focus and stop attending to your worries and distractions for a little while.

2. **Exercise.** Research tells us that regular exercise can help reduce symptoms of anxiety. So go for a walk or a run, dust off that soccer (fútbol) and start juggling, do some sit-ups, or have a dance party!

3. **Get good sleep.** We know from clinical studies that young people who don't get more or high-quality sleep report higher symptoms of anxiety and lack of concentration. You can set a bedtime alarm, track your sleep with an app, or set a regular bedtime and stick to it for a week. Whatever you choose, do what you can to get at least seven to eight hours a night.

4. **Reduce stress.** Lower stress exposure and stress management help us reduce our potential for developing an anxiety disorder. (Check out Mindset 5 for more on stress.)

5. **Engage in positive cultural practices.** It's important for young people with marginalized identities to understand how anxiety can be triggered by exposure to discrimination. Thankfully, focusing on the strength, beauty, and rich cultural practices of people from backgrounds like yours can help you manage the mental spin. Talk to your elders and other

supportive, wise folks who've been around long enough to recognize that we're a lot bigger and brighter than the challenges we've encountered.

🔍 JOURNAL PROMPT

Which of the suggestions for helping yourself lit you up the most? Why? In what ways can you start incorporating them into your life to boost your mood, hone your focus, and be more present and peaceful?

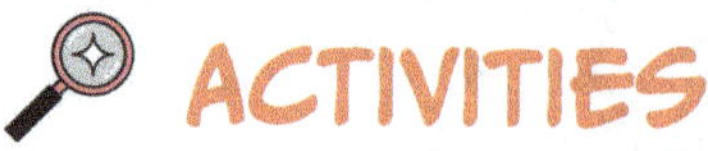

ACTIVITIES

Now that you know something about anxiety and coping strategies, let's practice some new skills.

EASY

Positive Affirmation

Find a quiet place to sit, preferably on the ground (it's OK, you can even place a towel or blanket under you if you hate bugs and crawly things). Then, open your camera app. Take two to three deep breaths, and record a video of yourself saying the following, slowly and with care:

I have worries, but worries don't have me.

Save your recording on your device. Whenever you need to stop feeding the fear and start feeding your power, go back to that video and pay attention to how it feels in your body to hear yourself say those words.

After this activity, I feel:

MINDSET 2

MODERATE

Talk to a Loved One About Anxiety

First, open a browser or dictionary and look up "anxiety." Then, write down a definition that makes sense to you: not just the technical words but how you might explain it to a friend.

Next, think about someone in your family—or your found family (chosen family, friends, mentors, etc.). who you think might understand what anxiety feels like. Pick someone you feel safe talking to.

When you're ready, ask them if they'd be OK with you asking a couple questions. You can say something like, "I'm learning about anxiety for myself, and I'm wondering if you've ever felt it. Could I ask you a couple questions?"

Here are two you can start with:

1. What is your earliest memory of feeling anxious?
2. Did anyone talk to you about anxiety and how to deal with it when you were younger?
3. (Optional: You can create your own third question, especially if there's something you've been wondering, like—*Do you ever feel like you're the only one going through this?* or *What helps you feel calmer when you're overwhelmed?*)

Just remember to be curious but not pushy; you're opening a door, not digging for secrets.

After you talk to them, take a quiet moment to think about what they said. Were there any surprises or "I can relate" moments?

Every time you slow down to notice, reflect, and connect, you're strengthening your focus muscle, which helps you stay grounded when things feel stormy. And maybe, most importantly, you've just taken a step toward normalizing something that is often hidden away. Remember, anxiety isn't a flaw. It's a signal that can run in families and social groups: through genetics, through stress, and through silence.

After this activity, I feel:

HARD

Slow Down and Breathe Deep

This breathing activity is labeled "hard" not because the steps are complicated, but because it asks something that can *feel* challenging: to slow down
and focus. That can be tough, especially if you're used to always being in
motion or distracted. The challenge isn't the task itself—it's the shift in
behavior. Learning to do something differently, especially when it involves
stillness and awareness, takes practice and patience.

Center yourself by finding a quiet space. Once you're comfortable,
intentionally push your shoulders down toward the ground to release
tension.

Next, take a deep breath in and blow it out. Aim to breathe in for four
seconds and hold for two; then, breathe out for four seconds and hold for
two (this is known as box breathing).

Now, see if you can breathe in for ten full cycles of breath (inhale for
four seconds, hold for two, exhale four seconds, hold for two).

Afterward, notice how you feel. Do you feel the same as you did when
you started this exercise, or different?

This simple grounding and breathing exercise absolutely forces us to
focus our energy on being present. Also, when we slow down our breathing,
we practice grace (i.e., patient loving kindness) and give ourselves respite,

which literally activates our parasympathetic nervous system's (i.e. the part of your nervous system focused on rest, recovery, and relation among other things) relaxation response (and feels *really* good!).

After this activity, I feel:

🔍 KEY TAKEAWAYS

Congrats! You made it to the end of Mindset 2: May the Focus Be with You! Have you learned anything you want to incorporate into your daily routine? Is there anything in this section you want to shout from the rooftops about? Maybe you've learned something you can share with your friends or parents/caregivers to help them. Make a note of your key takeaways (including the ones you'd like to share with others) and write them below:

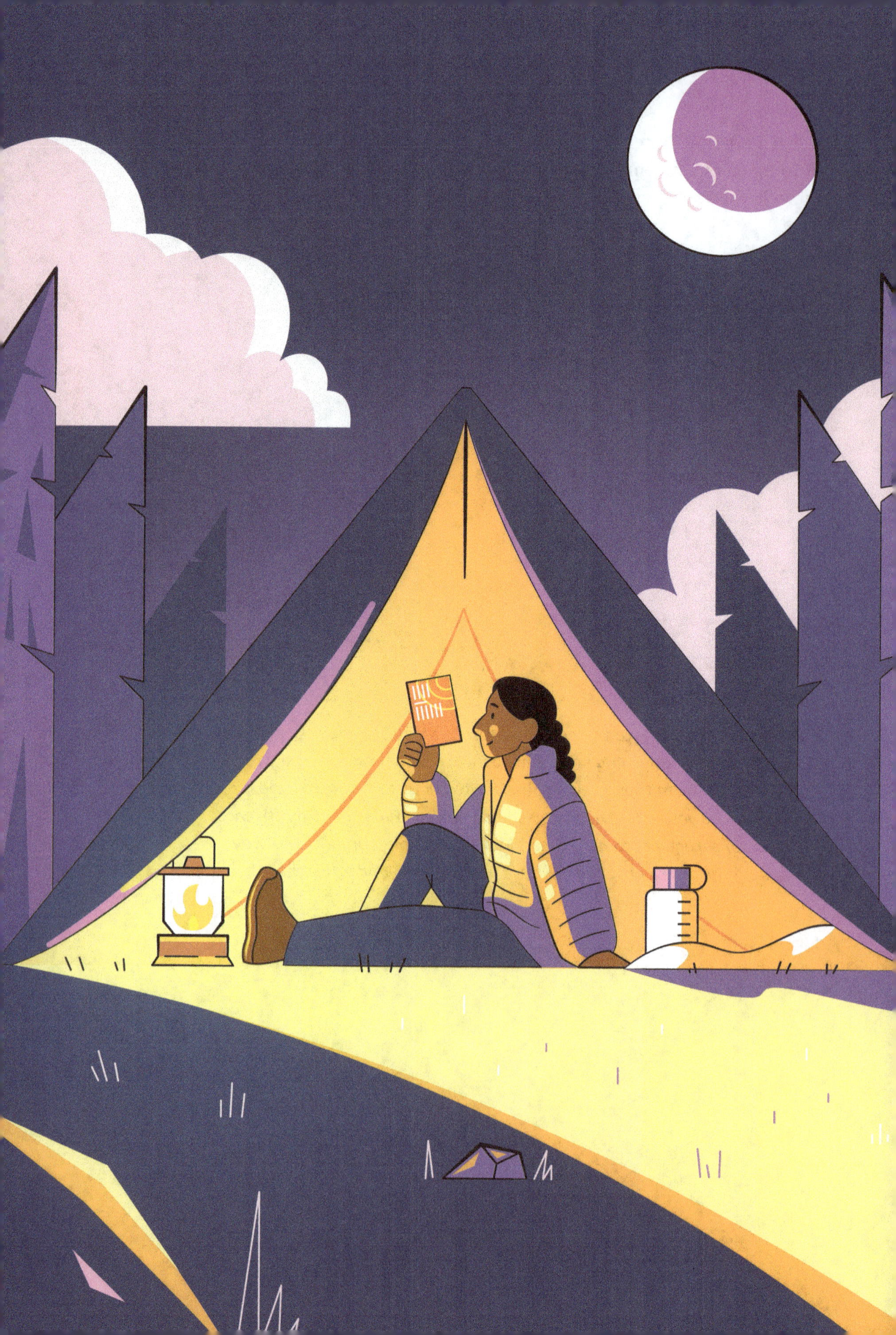

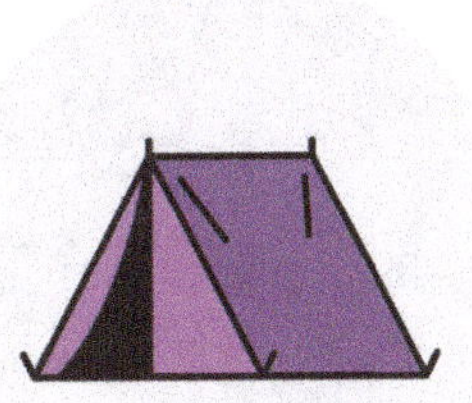

Hold Space 4 U

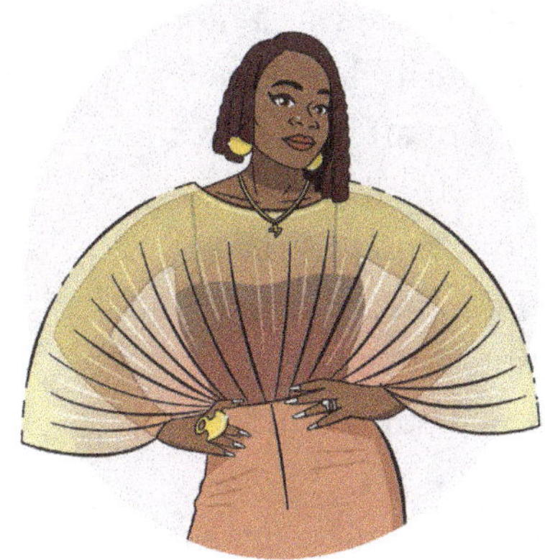

Life can feel overwhelming, especially in a world that often makes us feel like we're not enough or that our feelings don't matter. But learning to "hold space" for yourself—being kind to yourself, recognizing your emotions, and not letting the outside world decide your worth—is one of the most important things you can do for your mental health. When we ignore our feelings or rely too much on what others think of us, it can make us feel lost, anxious, or even depressed. But when we create a safe space inside ourselves, we build confidence, self-respect, and emotional strength. We can use this mindset as a weapon to fight the symptoms of depression and make it a bit easier to get through tough times.

By the end of this section, you will know more about:

- Depressive illness (we commonly call it depression)
- Depression vs. run-of-the-mill sadness
- Signs and symptoms of depression
- Why "holding space" for yourself is important
- When to seek help
- Navigating suicidal thoughts

Let's Get Started

Back when I was still a psychiatry professor—before I founded a nonprofit—I worked with all kinds of families. One that sticks with me was a mom and her teenage son, both African American. He was polite at first, showing up to our sessions, nodding along, keeping things cool. But after just a few visits, something changed.

One day, they arrived, and he flat-out refused to come into my office. The front desk called me out to the lobby, and when I got there, he was going off—yelling, stomping, and making it clear he wasn't coming in for therapy. Then, before anyone could stop him, he stormed out the front doors, ignoring his mom as she called after him.

I could see that his mom was shaken, embarrassed. So I took a deep breath, asked her to take a seat, and then walked outside after him. I didn't chase him. I just followed, about fifteen to twenty steps behind, listening as he vented. After a moment, I calmly called his name.

And just like that, he stopped mid-yell. He turned around, looked at me, and—respectfully, like a completely different person—said, "Yes, ma'am?" Then, without a fight, he followed me back inside. We sat down, and he was respectful the whole session.

So what was the big deal? It turned out he was upset because his hair wasn't freshly cut before coming to therapy. He felt ashamed of stepping out of the house not looking his best. That was it.

And here's why this story matters: Depression doesn't always show up as sadness. Sometimes, it looks like anger. Like shutting down. Like lashing out. It can disguise itself as things people misunderstand—bad moods, attitude, disrespect. But underneath, it's pain.

The key is to recognize it when it creeps in and learn how to walk through it—so it doesn't take over your life.

Our goal? To take up so much space—mentally, emotionally, physically—that depression has no choice but to shrink. Keep reading to learn how to do just that.

 # What Is Depression?

When you think of depression, what comes to mind? Someone curled up in bed, covers pulled over their head, not wanting to face the world? Yeah, that can be part of it—but it's not the whole picture.

According to the *Diagnostic and Statistical Manual of Mental Disorders, 5th Edition, Text Revision* (DSM-5-TR), depression is defined as "a mood disorder that involves persistent sadness and loss of interest."[5] But let's be real—depression isn't just about feeling sad. It's an illness that affects your whole self—emotionally, physically, and even spiritually.

A lot of people wear masks to cover their depression. Why? Because they feel ashamed that they can't just "snap out of it." Maybe they grew up in families where parents or caregivers brushed off their feelings—saying things like, "You're so young, what do you have to be sad about?" (Then immediately launching into a rant about their own problems.)

I get it. I've been there myself. In my early twenties, after a really traumatic experience, I went through clinical depression. I know exactly how hard it can be to cope—how it feels when the world tells you to just *keep going* when all you want to do is curl up in bed and cry.

And here's what you need to know:

- Depression is the number one reason people miss work and school worldwide.
- In the U.S., about 15–20% of all young people under eighteen experience depression.[6]
- In 2025, my nonprofit, The AAKOMA Project, found that over 63% of young people from diverse backgrounds said they've experienced moderate to severe depression since the pandemic.[7]

5. American Psychiatric Association. *Diagnostic and Statistical Manual of Mental Disorders*, 5th ed., text rev. (Arlington, VA: American Psychiatric Association, 2022). https://doi.org/10.1176/appi. books.9780890425787.

6. Wilson, S., and N. M. Dumornay. "Rising Rates of Adolescent Depression in the United States: Challenges and Opportunities in the 2020s." Journal of Adolescent Health 70, no. 3 (March 2022): 354–55. https://doi.org/10.1016/j.jadohealth.2021.12.003.

7. Breland-Noble, A., The AAKOMA Project, and C. A. Harb. *State of Mental Health of Youth and Young Adults of Color, Full Report.* 2025.

Depression makes you feel like you need to hide from the world. Like you need to withdraw and hold yourself back. But I want you to hear me  when I say: That is depression talking. That is not you. Your best self is still in there, waiting to be heard. Keep reading to learn more about depression—how to spot it, how it shows up in unexpected ways, and what you can do to fight back. And be sure to check out the video through this QR code—in it, I share surprising ways depression can show up.

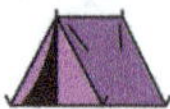 # JOURNAL PROMPT

When you hear the word depression, what comes to mind? What conversations have you had with people you love and respect about depression? What have you seen in the media about depression? How have you seen it discussed in your own community, family, or culture? Do you feel media portrayals show something different from what you've learned in your family or community? Which conversations (media or family/culture) reflect your own understanding of depression? Can you describe how?

Signs and Symptoms of Depression

The best way to spot depression? Pay attention to how you feel day to day, then compare it to how you've felt over the past week or two. If you notice any of the following signs sticking around, it might be more than just a bad mood:

 Feeling sad or low most of the time

 Uncontrollable crying, even when you don't know why

 Losing interest in things you usually love (like gaming, texting with friends, or your art)

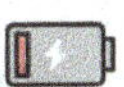 Low energy multiple times a week, even when you're getting enough rest

 Struggling to sleep—or sleeping way more than usual

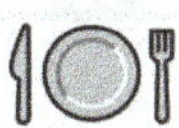 Losing your appetite—or eating way more than normal

But here's something people don't talk about enough—depression in teens doesn't always look like sadness. I wrote a chapter in a book about youth depression, and we talked about some less obvious symptoms that often show up in young people:

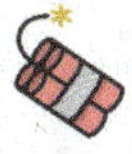 Irritability—feeling annoyed by <u>everything</u>

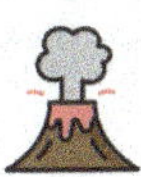 Anger & outbursts—getting mad more easily than usual

 Doing worse in school—losing focus, struggling with motivation, or just not caring anymore

For depression to be diagnosed, these changes usually need to stick around for at least two weeks and feel like a big shift from what's normal for you. If this sounds familiar, keep reading—there's help, and you don't have to deal with this alone.

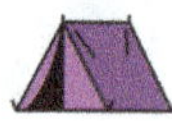 # JOURNAL PROMPT

Think about a time when you felt a deep sadness, numbness, or heaviness—whether you named it depression or not. What did it feel like in your body? What thoughts ran through your mind? How did it shape the way you showed up in the world? Did you act differently than you would have otherwise? Now, go a bit deeper: What do you think the sadness, numbness, and heaviness were asking of you? Were they seeking rest, asking you to change something in your environment, asking you to change the way you connect to other people? If your depression could talk to you, kindly but directly, what would it say? And if you could respond to it with kindness and compassion, what would you say?

Don't Hide Your Shine!

Depression lies. It tries to convince you that you're not worthy, that you're not enough, that you should feel ashamed or guilty for what you're experiencing. It tells you to stay small, to disappear, to keep your struggles hidden.

Let me make something very clear: You are worthy. You are enough. And there is nothing about who you are as a person to be ashamed of.

Think of your mind like it has built-in noise cancellation—you have the power to tune out the lies that depression feeds you. It might tell you to make yourself smaller, to stay quiet so others don't notice your pain, to withdraw so you won't be hurt. That instinct—to shrink and protect yourself—can feel like the only way to cope.

But there is a better way.

Too often, people with marginalized identities are pressured to blend in, to avoid drawing attention, to keep the peace at all costs. We're told that if we stay quiet, if we don't make waves, life will somehow be easier—that if we just go along with things, everything will be OK. But that is simply not true. When we "go along to get along," we go against ourselves.

Each of us has that *knowing* inside—a gut feeling, an inner voice that tells us when something isn't right. Some call it a moral compass, others call it intuition, but whatever name it takes, it belongs to *you* alone. When we allow others to dictate how we think, feel, or act, we silence that voice, and our bodies, minds, and spirits don't let it slide. The signs are always there—a sudden stomach ache, a tightness in the chest, a pause that stops you in your tracks. If we pay attention, we *always* know when we are betraying ourselves.

My grandmother on my mom's side taught me something simple but powerful: "Follow your first mind." That means listening to your inner voice, the one that quietly but clearly points you in the right direction. Because when we ignore it just to keep others comfortable, we begin to lose touch with ourselves. And self-alienation—the feeling of being disconnected from who we really are—is a key feature of depression.

Staying quiet doesn't make things better—it only makes *you* feel invisible. It keeps you from getting the support you deserve. You don't have to silence yourself to survive. You don't have to disappear to protect yourself. You *deserve* to take up space.

You take up space by refusing to self-silence. By voicing your opinion even when it's unpopular. By making your own thoughtful decisions and standing by them, even when others disagree. Sometimes you take up space in quieter ways—by wearing your hair in a style that reflects your culture, by bringing your favorite home-cooked meal to lunch and not apologizing for its scent, by embracing your unique style of dress or the accent that makes your voice distinct. Taking up space means refusing to let others make you feel small.

I have always told my own children: "Never call someone else weird or different because we are all different from each other." We don't use labels to ostracize people, and we don't let others use words like *weird* or accusations of *doing too much* or *being extra* to make someone shrink. You deserve to be seen, to be heard, to be exactly who you are—without apology.

Depression convinces us we *should* shrink. It tells us that staying small, withdrawing, and fading into the background will keep us from getting hurt. It whispers that avoiding vulnerability is safer. That's a lie. The sooner we recognize the warning signs—the exhaustion, the sadness, the hopelessness—the sooner we can push back. Active coping won't magically erase struggle, but it *can* loosen the grip of depression before it tightens. And if you're already deep in it, it can help you claw your way out.

You are not here to disappear. You are here to *be*. So don't shrink to make anyone comfortable—no matter what.

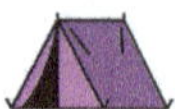 JOURNAL PROMPT

Think about a time when you made yourself smaller—whether by staying quiet, downplaying your identity, or hiding (staying in the background, fading to the back of the room)—to protect yourself from harm or to reduce other people's discomfort. What did that moment feel like for you? In your body? In your mind? In your heart? What emotions surfaced? Do you feel that it helped you in the moment? Now, consider this. There is a deeper cost to shrinking yourself: What parts of yourself did you hide or sacrifice in that moment? What would it feel like to not hide or sacrifice? To take up the space you deserve, even in places where your identity is underrepresented? What would you need—within yourself and from others—to feel safe taking up the space you deserve?

MINDSET 3

When Depression Becomes Despair

If we let depression run unchecked, it doesn't just sit still—it grows. It picks up speed, like a snowball rolling downhill, except instead of gaining positive momentum, it spirals downward, leaving sadness, chaos, and destruction in its path. And if we don't actively work to cope, to care for ourselves, to fight back, depression can lead to something even heavier: despair.

Despair is what happens when depression goes on for so long, unchecked, that it starts to feel like there's no way out. It's when the weight of everything becomes unbearable, when hopelessness settles in, when you start believing—wrongly—that nothing will ever get better. It's a dangerous place to be because it can lead to suicidal thoughts. And unfortunately, this is something far too many young people experience today. In our SOMHYOC 2025 data, We found that a whopping 83% of all Youth of Color surveyed reported experiencing any symptoms of depression, with 60% of youth in our study reporting experiencing moderate to severe depression.[8]

As it relates to suicidal thoughts (also known as suicidal ideation), 37% of the diverse youth asked in our study reported seriously considering suicide in the prior twelve months.[9]

Look around. We live in a world where people talk about the "loneliness epidemic"—where so many of us feel disconnected, unseen, unheard. We scroll through perfect-looking lives on social media while struggling with our own reality. We hear about rising rates of depression, about people feeling more isolated than ever. And when we're surrounded by others who are also struggling, it can start to feel normal to feel miserable. But just because something feels common doesn't mean it's OK.

Being around other people who are depressed can impact us. It can reinforce the idea that there's no way out, that suffering is just something

---

8. Breland-Noble, A., The AAKOMA Project, and C. A. Harb. *State of Mental Health of Youth and Young Adults of Color,* Full Report. 2025.
9. Ibid.

we have to endure. It can make us feel like our own pain is insignificant, or worse, that there's no hope for relief.

But there is hope. There are options.

For some, psychotherapy and lifestyle changes—like exercise, social connection, and mindfulness—can help. For others, medication is a necessary tool, not a weakness. Depression is an illness, and just like with any other illness, sometimes medical treatment is needed. If you had a broken leg, you wouldn't try to just "tough it out"—you'd go to a doctor, right? Depression deserves the same care.

The most important thing to remember is this: Despair lies, just like depression does. It makes you think you're out of options when, in reality, there are always paths forward.

If you're feeling stuck in that dark place, if you're having thoughts about not wanting to be here anymore, please tell someone. A friend, a family member, a counselor, a helpline. You don't have to fight this alone. You are not a burden. You deserve help. And even if you can't see it now, there is a future where you get to feel like yourself again.

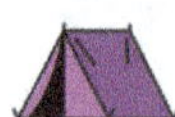

If you or anyone else you know might be struggling with depression or heavy thoughts, I want you to know you're not alone. I'm including a QR code here that links to a video about suicidal ideation—it's honest, compassionate, and might help you feel a little more seen and supported.

🏕️ JOURNAL PROMPT

Look around at the world today—how do you see despair taking shape in the people and communities around you, especially the communities you belong to? Have you ever felt the weight of someone else's depression settle onto your own shoulders? How did it affect you? Now, turn inward: When you have felt yourself sinking into heaviness, what helped (or didn't help) you find your way back? If despair is a descent, what might be the handholds—big or small—that can slow the fall or help in climbing back up?

I Have Depression—How Do I Help Myself?

I know what depression feels like—not just a passing bad mood, but the kind that makes everything feel impossible. The kind where getting out of bed feels like lifting a 150-pound weight. The kind that makes you wonder, *What's the point?* But you push through anyway, because you feel like you *have* to—because people are counting on you. Your friends, your parents, your siblings, your teammates. So you tell yourself you must keep going, no matter how exhausted or empty you feel.

And then, on top of everything, there are the messages we hear from people who mean well: "We're strong. We don't hide from our problems, we face them head-on."

"You're just a kid—what do you even have to be stressed about?"

These words might be meant to help, but all they really do is make us feel like we have no other option but to "suck it up" and deal with it alone. But I am here to ask you, to beg you—please don't go down that road.

This book is designed to help you avoid that trap—the fear-based thinking that tells you there are only two choices: push through or give up. That's not how the world works. That kind of thinking makes you feel powerless, like you don't know yourself, like you aren't capable of deciding what's best for you. But that's not true. There are billions of people in this world, which means there are billions of ways to approach a problem—including yours.

You deserve better than what depression is telling you right now. If you can carve out just five minutes a day to focus on learning coping skills, those five minutes can turn into weeks, then months, then years of actively managing your mental health. And not just in some vague, abstract way—I'm talking about real, science-backed, culturally relevant strategies that actually work.

Let's talk about how you can start managing depression in a way that works for you.

1. **Name your experience.** Remember Mindset 1? You can't fight something if you don't acknowledge it. So take a moment and name what you're feeling. Are you sad most of the time? Crying often? Feeling irritable or short-tempered? Are you exhausted no matter how much you sleep? Have you lost interest in things you used to love? How long have you felt this way? If it's been more than two weeks, this isn't just a rough patch. It's something that deserves attention. Once you name it, you can start taking steps to cope.

2. **Do some research about depression.** You deserve to understand what's happening to you. Learn about depression—what the symptoms are, what causes it, and how many people struggle with it. Knowing you're not alone can make a huge difference. In my 2025 SOMHYOC study, we found that 60.2% of Youth and Young Adults of Color reported experiencing moderate to severe depression in the past week.[10] The most common symptom? Little to no interest in doing things they once loved. If you've lost your spark and it's been a few weeks since you've seen it, it might be time to reach out for help.

3. **No more beating yourself up.** Let's stop tearing ourselves down for "failing" and start praising ourselves for trying. I always say, we either learn, or we grow. There is no failure— only lessons.

4. **Talk to someone you trust.** Talking about what you're going through is one of the most powerful things you can do. In our SOMHYOC 2025 study, young people told us that when they have a mental-health concern, they are most likely to talk to parents or caregivers, friends, or another trusted adult (a teacher, coach, mentor, etc.).[11] It doesn't matter who you open up to—what matters is that you don't keep it bottled up.

---

10. Breland-Noble, A., The AAKOMA Project, and C. A. Harb. *State of Mental Health of Youth and Young Adults of Color, Full Report.* 2025.
11. Ibid.

5. **Practice contemplative reflection.** This is just a fancy way of saying "sit with yourself and let your thoughts flow without judgment." You may have heard it called mindfulness, meditation, or breathwork. It doesn't have to be complicated. Just:

   - Find a quiet space.
   - Take a few deep breaths.
   - Let your thoughts drift in and out without attaching meaning to them.

Depression can feel like a thick fog—it clouds everything, making it hard to think clearly. Even a few moments of stillness can help cut through that fog, even if just a little.

I know that depression can make it feel like this is just *your life now*. Like you'll always feel this way. But that's not true. Small steps lead to big changes—and the fact that you're here, reading this, means you're already taking those first steps.

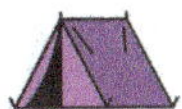 ## JOURNAL PROMPT

Which of the suggestions for helping yourself lit you up the most? Why? In what ways can you start incorporating them into your life to lift up your mood when you are down, and to help you remember to never shrink yourself?

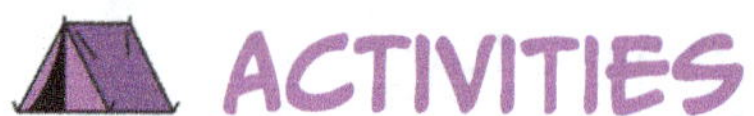 ## ACTIVITIES

Now that you know something about depression and coping strategies, let's practice some new skills.

EASY

One-Week Media Detox

For one week, I want you to pay attention to what you're feeding your brain. That means stepping away from any media—books, TV shows, podcasts, social media, YouTube, music, or movies—that doesn't uplift you. If it's heavy, dark, stressful, or makes you feel drained, press pause on it.

I know this might sound extreme, but think about it. What we consume affects how we feel. If you're constantly watching crime shows, listening to true crime podcasts, doomscrolling through bad news, or even just following people online who make you feel like you're not enough, that seeps into your mind. It shapes how you see the world and how you feel about yourself.

This doesn't mean you can never watch or listen to these things again—just take a break for one week. If you're as obsessed with *Law & Order* as I am, that means stepping away from it for seven days. If you always have a murder mystery podcast playing in the background, swap it for something lighter. If your TikTok feed is full of people ranting, fighting, or posting depressing content, give yourself permission to mute, unfollow, or just take a break.

At the end of the week, check in with yourself. How did it feel to not have those images, sounds, and stories constantly in your head? Did you feel lighter? Less anxious? More present in your own life? Did you notice a difference in your mood? You might be surprised at how much your mental state shifts just by being intentional about what you let into your mind. Give it a try.

After this activity, I feel:

____

____

____

____

____

MODERATE

Hit Mute and Reclaim Your Mind

Social media shapes how we see ourselves, often without us even realizing it. For the next fourteen days, try this simple experiment:

1. Pick your two most-used social media apps.
2. Mute the three influencers you pay the most attention to.
3. Stay off their content—no peeking!

That's it. No unfollowing, just a break. Why? Because constantly seeing someone else's highlight reel can make us feel like we're not doing enough, not successful enough, not *enough*. This isn't about them—it's about giving yourself space to think, feel, and exist without comparison.

At the end of fourteen days, journal about it. Did you miss them? Did you feel freer? Less pressure? More in tune with your own life? If you noticed a positive change, you get to decide what happens next.

After this activity, I feel:

HARD

See Yourself through the Eyes of Love

Sometimes, we're our own worst critics. We focus on what we think we're lacking instead of seeing ourselves the way the people who love us do. For the next month, try this simple practice to remind yourself of who you really are.

1. Grab a paper wall calendar—no phones, no apps, just something physical you can see every day.
2. Think of the five compliments you hear most from the people in your life.
3. Write them down in the language you learned them in (if your grandmother tells you in Tigrinya, write it in Tigrinya).
4. Each morning, use different-colored markers to write one of those compliments under the day's date.

That's it. Just a moment, first thing in the morning, to remind yourself that someone who truly knows you sees this in you. That means it's real—it's part of who you are. At the end of the month, look back at those words. Let them sink in. Because no matter what your mind tells you on hard days, this is the truth about you.

After this activity, I feel:

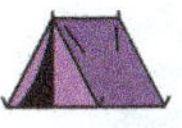 # KEY TAKEAWAYS

Congrats! You made it to the end of Mindset 3: Hold Space 4 U! Have you learned anything you want to incorporate into your daily routine? Is there anything in this section you want to shout from the rooftops about? Maybe you've learned something you can share with your friends or parents/ caregivers to help them. Make a note of your key takeaways (including the ones you'd like to share with others) and write them below:

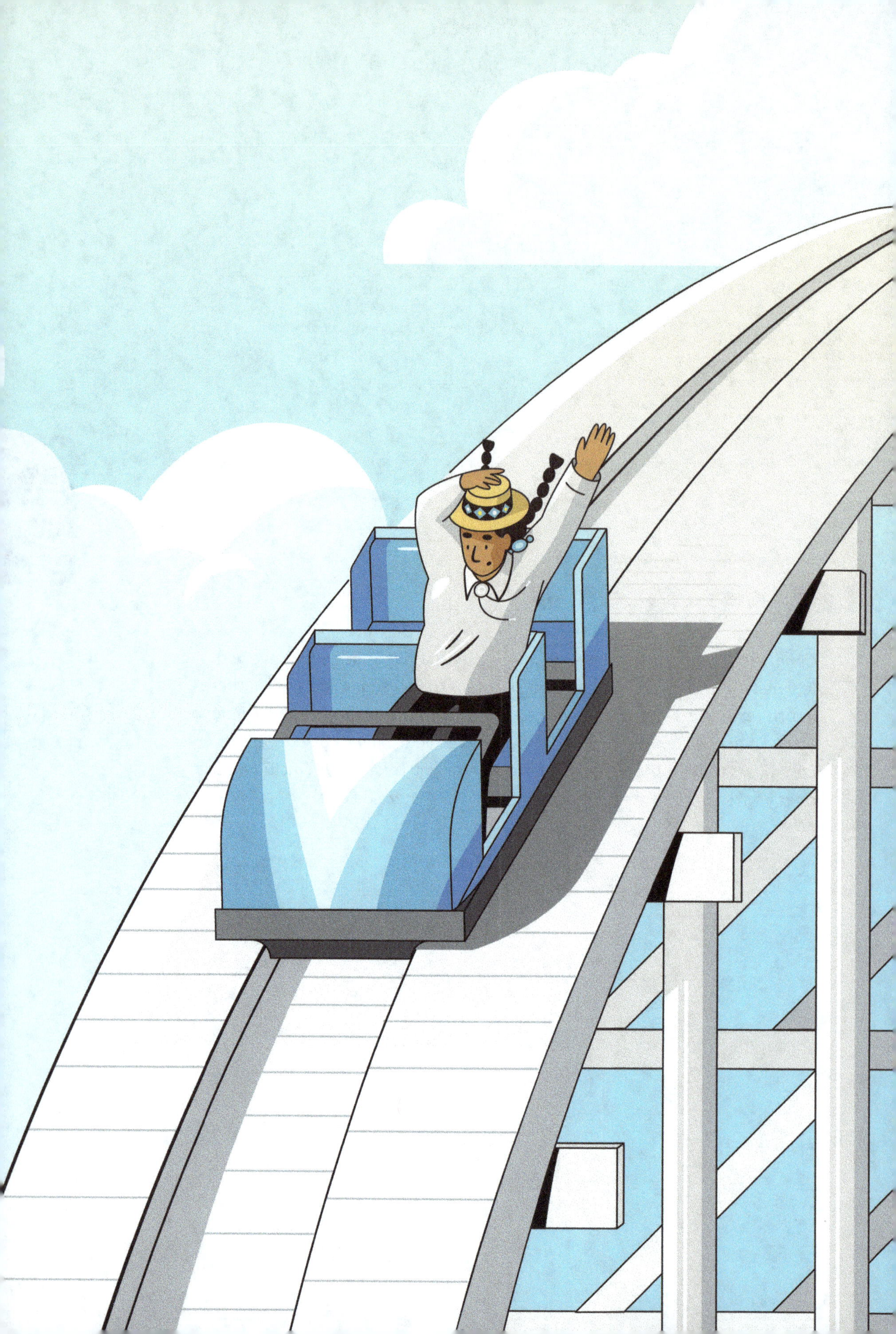

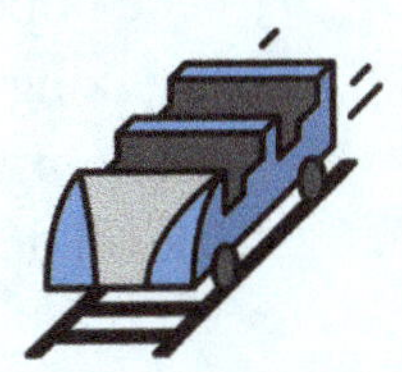

Mindset 4

Ride the Roller Coaster

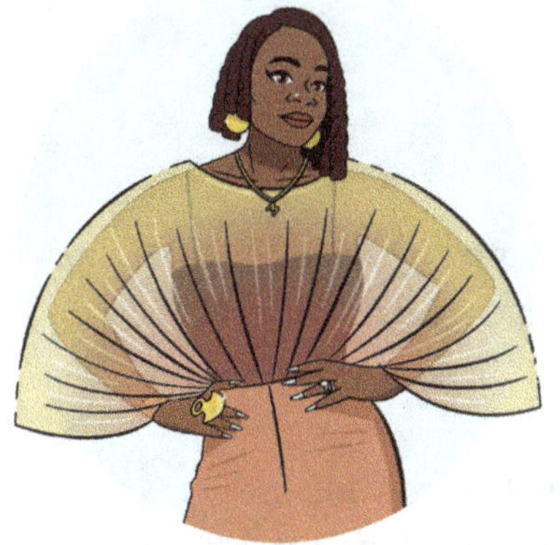

Life can feel like a never-ending roller coaster—one moment you're soaring, the next you're plummeting, and sometimes you're just stuck upside down wondering how you even got there. Emotions can be wild like that. One second you're chilling, and the next, you're overwhelmed by a wave of feelings you didn't even see coming. Totally normal.

The good news? You don't have to just hang on for dear life. You have more control than you think! When emotions start to take over—whether it's stress, excitement, frustration, or that weird mix of everything at once—you can learn to navigate that roller coaster with self-compassion instead of letting them throw you around.

Think of this as your emotional "control panel." In this section, we'll break down what's happening inside you when emotions get intense, why it's completely OK to feel big feelings, and, most importantly, how to ride the waves without getting wiped out.

By the end of this section, you will know more about:

- Why ups and downs are a normal part of being human (and why all emotions are totally valid, even if they're not accurate)
- How to find your neutral heart space when you're not grounded
- What emotional regulation and dysregulation are—and how you can feel them in your body

- The importance of understanding our negative automatic thinking
- Defining conditions with big feelings (bipolar disorder, oppositional defiant disorder)

Let's Get Started

There was a boy, about ten years old, who'd been adopted by a couple—one parent shared his background, the other didn't. His dad worked a lot. His mom stayed home but was often exhausted. He didn't have any brothers or sisters, and, most days, he felt alone.

Even though he was bright, school was tough. He kept getting in trouble. He lost friends easily. At home, things weren't much better. He was acting out in ways he couldn't explain, and it started to feel like everyone—his teachers, his parents, even the kids at school—saw him as the problem.

That's when he and his family came to see me. I worked with him for a few months and got to know the weight he was carrying. His dad was always busy. His mom was burnt out. He didn't feel seen. He told me more than once that he felt like a burden, like just *being* was too much for his family.

Then, one day, his mom showed up to our session alone. She was panicked. Her son had disappeared. No one at school knew where he was. She hadn't called the police—she was too ashamed—but we were all trying to stay calm and figure out where he might've gone.

Almost an hour later, she drove home—and there he was, sitting on the front porch, waiting. He had taken the city bus by himself, made a few transfers, and quietly made his way home. He hadn't told anyone. He didn't run away. He just . . . didn't want to come to therapy that day. He said he was tired of everything being focused on him. It made him feel like he was broken, like the only one who needed fixing.

And honestly? That made sense. He was struggling—not because he was bad or wrong, but because he felt out of place. He didn't know how to express what he was feeling, and he didn't have a safe outlet to let those feelings move through. Over time, he started to believe the story the world was telling him: *You're too much. You're the problem.*

But here's what I want you to know (and that I so badly wished that young boy knew): Just because you're feeling lost, angry, overwhelmed, or misunderstood—it doesn't mean *you* are the problem. You're human.

You're allowed to feel big things. You're allowed to not know what to do with them sometimes. That doesn't make you broken. That makes you real.

The road back to yourself isn't about being perfect or figuring it all out overnight. It's about learning how to ride the emotional waves, how to honor what's true for you, and how to keep coming back to your center—your baseline—again and again.

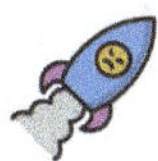 What Does "Out of Control" Feel Like . . . and How Do We Get to Baseline?

The little boy in the story had a lot of big feelings, many of them quite understandable. It was his behavior in response to those big feelings that got him into difficult situations. I used to tell him, and I say to you today, your feelings are 100 percent VALID. If you feel it, it matters. No one has the right to tell you otherwise. But here's the tricky part—sometimes, feelings lie. Sometimes, they grab the mic, crank up the volume, and convince you that one bad moment is the end of the world. And when that happens, when you're caught in the middle of a full-on emotional hurricane, it's easy to believe that there's no way out.

It starts small. You wake up with a plan. You know exactly what you're going to wear, how you're going to look, the way you're going to step into the world that day. And then—disaster. The shoes you were counting on? Not there. The hair you spent hours perfecting? Betrayed you. Maybe it's a small thing, something other people might brush off, but for you, in that moment, it's everything. You can feel the shift, the way your heart sinks, the way your body tightens up. And suddenly, the thought sneaks in: *This whole day is ruined.* And just like that, the spiral begins.

It doesn't stop with one bad moment. It grows. *If my hair looks bad, everyone's going to notice. If everyone notices, they'll think I'm ugly. If they think I'm ugly, what's the point of even trying?* The feeling morphs into something bigger, stretching into places it doesn't belong, twisting into new fears and doubts. One thing goes wrong, and now it's not just about your hair or your shoes—it's about *you.* And that's when emotions have you. That's when they take the wheel and floor it straight toward catastrophe. In those moments, it is important for you to know that your brain is wired to experience things intensely. And that's OK. While your feelings are valid, they are not always precise and they are definitely not permanent..

The world isn't exactly built for emotional balance. Every day, you're hit with a constant flood of notifications, opinions, and expectations—social-media feeds packed with highlight reels, news cycles designed to spark outrage, text and group chats as part of your daily download, and a culture that rewards quick reactions over thoughtful responses. Especially for marginalized groups, including People of Color and all their intersections, LGBTQAI+ young people and those with disabilities, there are patterns we see popularized by others—ways of reacting, surviving, or shutting down—that we can confidently say would not work for us and that we do not want to carry forward.

Remember, *just because the world runs on chaos doesn't mean you have to.* You get to set your own tone and lead with your own clarity. And when you do, you give others permission to do the same. Instead of absorbing the stress and dysfunction around you, what if you chose to be the one who leads with calm? You are empowered to do better than what you see—you are empowered to thrive.

Now, is this easy and one-and-done? Absolutely not, because for many of us, conversations about mental health are limited to a feeling word chart on the wall of our kindergarten classroom. We are generally not taught to do anything other than recognize emotions. But what about managing them? We're so used to running, performing, and keeping up, we never stop to ask: *What do I feel like when I'm not reacting to something? Who am I when I'm not worried about how other people see me?*

Even in the midst of all the noise around you, I'm hoping that you can identify the space where everything is just . . . OK. Not amazing, not awful. Just neutral. That's your baseline. And if you don't know what it feels like, it's impossible to find your way back to it when emotional reactions knock you off balance.

Your baseline feels like easy breathing, little to no tension in your body, clarity of mind. That's what it's like to be in your neutral heart space. For so many, the challenge is finding those moments day to day—knowing when we feel it and knowing how to achieve it at any moment.

Here's what I want you to remember: Your feelings are valid, but they're not always precise.

In other words, while it is always important to acknowledge our feelings, it can be just as important to put them in context, to make sure that we are responding to the moment we are faced with, not the moment we have dreamed up in our heads.

So how do you do that?

You take time to notice. Notice when the spiraling *begins*. Notice when the story in your head is getting bigger than the reality in front of you. Notice what it feels like when you're *not* overwhelmed, so you can find your way back when you are.

You are not a machine, designed to "on" twenty-four seven. You're a person, a human. By definition, you need to pause. You are allowed to feel. And you must remember—no matter how big the emotions get, we can never allow them to control us. With the right support, we can *always* find and use tools to help us control our emotions and take back the wheel.

Check out the video using the QR code here—it'll shed more light on the differences between feeling in control and out of control.

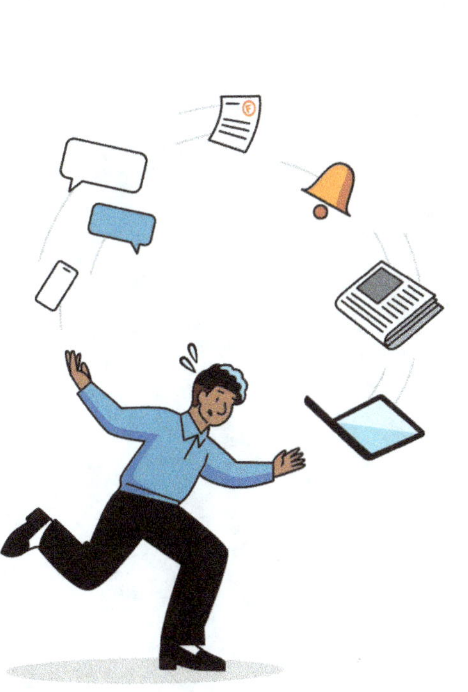
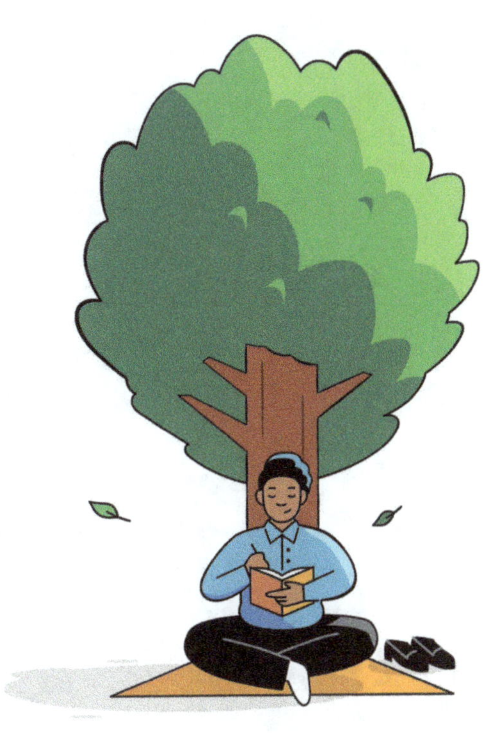

Feeling out of control vs. feeling in control

JOURNAL PROMPT

Think about a time when your emotions took over—when one bad moment turned into a bad day, a bad week, or maybe even a bad version of yourself. Write about that experience in detail. What happened? What was the trigger? Did the story in your head get bigger than what actually happened? Now, take a deep breath and imagine hitting pause in that moment. If you could go back, what would you say to yourself? Not to dismiss your feelings, but to remind yourself that they don't have to control everything. How would you comfort yourself? What's one thing you could have done to find your balance again?

MINDSET 4

Signs and Symptoms of Emotional Self-Regulation

We all experience emotions—big ones, small ones, and everything in between. *Emotional regulation* is the ability to manage those emotions in a way that helps you navigate life without getting completely overwhelmed or stuck. It doesn't mean you never feel sad, anxious, or angry—it just means you can <u>recognize</u> those feelings, <u>process</u> them, and <u>respond</u> in a way that works for you, not against you. Here's how you know when you're regulated and at your baseline:

 You can recognize what you're feeling without letting it define your whole day

 You know how to pause and breathe before reacting

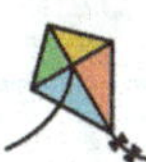 You can calm yourself down when emotions get intense

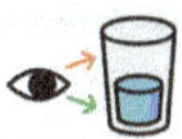 You're able to put things in perspective instead of catastrophizing

 You can communicate your feelings instead of shutting down or lashing out

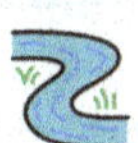 You allow yourself to feel emotions <u>without</u> letting them control your actions

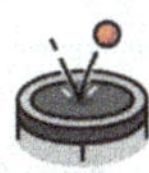 You bounce back after tough situations instead of staying stuck in them

 You know when to take a break and step away from overwhelming situations

 You can offer yourself kindness and self-compassion when you're struggling

 You understand that feelings <u>aren't facts</u>—just because something <u>feels</u> like the end of the world doesn't mean it actually is

Signs and Symptoms of Emotional Dysregulation

On the flip side, *emotional dysregulation* happens when emotions feel so intense that they take over, making it hard to think clearly, make decisions, or feel in control. It's when emotions <u>run the show</u>, and you feel like you're being dragged along for the ride instead of steering the wheel.

Here are some common signs:

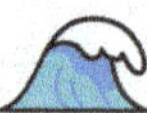 Your emotions feel <u>too big</u> to handle, like they're consuming you

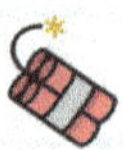 You react impulsively—saying or doing things before thinking them through

 Small things trigger extreme emotions (anger, sadness, anxiety, etc.)

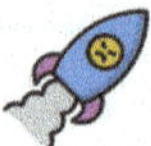 It's hard to calm down once you're upset—it feels like you're <u>stuck</u> there

 You avoid emotions by numbing out (scrolling, binge-watching, overworking, etc.)

 You feel overwhelmed by your feelings and don't know how to process them

 You have trouble expressing emotions in a way that others understand

 You dwell on the past or obsess over the future instead of staying present

 You get stuck in negative thought loops and struggle to break free

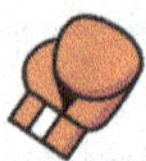 You beat yourself up for feeling emotional instead of giving yourself grace

Keep in mind that no one is <u>always</u> regulated or <u>always</u> dysregulated—it's a spectrum, and we all move along it depending on the situation. But the more you recognize where you are, the more power you have to shift yourself back into balance when emotions start pulling you off course.

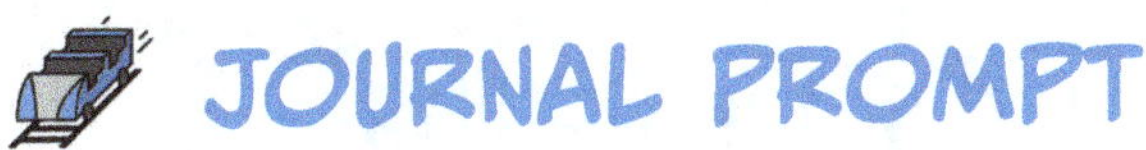 # JOURNAL PROMPT

Think of a time when you felt in control of your emotions—steady, clear-headed, able to handle whatever came your way. What was different about that moment? What did your body feel like? How did your thoughts sound?

Now, think of a time when your emotions took over—when you felt like a passenger on a runaway train. What set it off? What did it feel like in your body? If your emotions had a voice in that moment, what would they have said? Did the situation really deserve that level of intensity, or did it feel bigger than it was?

Looking at both moments, what do you notice? What pulls you off track? What helps you stay steady? If you could name one thing that brings you back to balance, what would it be? Write it down. Hold onto it. Next time overpowering emotions try to take the wheel, remember—you do know how to drive.

Overwhelm, Overloads, and Saying No! to Everything: Let's Talk About BPD and ODD

OK, so we already know emotions can be intense. Especially when you're growing up and your brain, your body, and your life are changing all the time. But sometimes, what looks like "moodiness" or "being headstrong" can actually be something deeper that deserves real attention, support, and understanding.

Let's break down two mental-health conditions that can seriously shake up day-to-day life for young people: **Bipolar Disorder (BPD)** and **Oppositional Defiant Disorder (ODD)**.

First up: Bipolar Disorder (aka the roller coaster). Think about BPD as a monster roller coaster, big ups and big downs. When I was a kid, there was this roller coaster at Busch Gardens in Williamsburg called the Loch Ness Monster. It was, for its time, a beast of a roller coaster and it's a perfect analogy for explaining BPD. BPD includes two extremes of emotions: First, there is the climb up—like on the Loch Ness, when the carriage slowly climbs up at an almost ninety-degree angle to a *really* high peak, and your mood is super high and you feel like you can do anything and may often try to do everything all at once (a state known as mania). Then there's the precipitous drop—on the Loch Ness, the one and only time I rode it, we careened down that almost ninety-degree angle at a hundred miles an hour, wind whipping through our hair, completely out of control. And I was terrified. That's what the drop of depression, which is the other side of BPD, can feel like: You're out of control, unable to get a handle on how you're feeling, sometimes stuck in feeling sad and, at times, even forlorn.

That's BPD, where emotional extremes are way more intense and disruptive than the usual highs and lows of life.

Here's what we've learned from years of research and working with families:

- BPD is usually diagnosed in the late teen years, because it takes time to tell the difference between typical teenage stuff and something more serious.
- Even though it's diagnosed later, early signs often show up in childhood—like super-intense mood swings or epic meltdowns.

- People with BPD often deal with unstable emotions, impulsive behavior (doing stuff without thinking it through), feeling bad about themselves, and having relationships that feel like emotional roller coasters.

BPD doesn't mean you're intentionally dramatic or "too much." However, it's a good idea to remember and understand that our genes, our brain chemistry, and our environments all impact us, and we need real tools and support to navigate the experience of BPD.

Now, let's talk about ODD (aka "I don't want to, and you can't make me"). You'll know when you experience someone with ODD because it feels like A LOT more than just a "no." An ODD no is not just regular teenage backtalk or slamming the bedroom door. An ODD no is BIG and is directed at everyone in authority, whether it's a teacher, parent/caregiver, or a friend; the words and the behaviors from someone with ODD are generally a big, fiery NO.

And here's what those giant NOs might look like:

- Constant arguing or refusing to follow rules
- Picking fights just to pick them
- Regularly trying to push people's buttons
- Getting stuck in patterns of anger, irritability, or defiance

And here's the part that warrants your attention: People with ODD usually don't see it in themselves. It's more about how others experience them. When you experience a person with ODD, you might find yourself saying, "Why does it always feel like I'm fighting with this person?" or "Why do they make even the smallest things feel like a tug of war?"

What's really going on?

Often, a person with ODD is not seeking attention; they are seeking acknowledgment. It's like their brain and whole body are saying: "I need you to see me. I need you to know I exist. I'm not invisible. I matter."

And none of that is bad or shameful. It's human. But if our experience is one of constant conflict or defiance, it might be time to pause and ask:

- Am I always fighting with the same person?
- Do I feel like no matter what I do, they're on my case?
- Are they being unfair—or am I reacting in a way that makes things worse?

And sometimes, the pattern is about the dynamic *between* people, not just the *behavior* of one person.

So in these instances, how do you find peace and equilibrium? You can start by learning to ride the waves of your emotions without getting knocked over. Practice naming what you feel, even when it feels messy or complicated. Use that wisdom to then help you learn what triggers that automatic NO!, then lean into figuring out how to use a smaller no when it's OK to say no—and when it might actually help to say yes.

And if your emotions or behavior are making life harder than it needs to be, you're not a problem, and you are not broken. You just need some support and new tools. And that's where self-reflection and psychotherapy can help you, because you deserve support, not shame. You're not just "a moody kid" or "a difficult, headstrong person." You're a whole human being who deserves to be seen and understood in a world that doesn't always make that easy.

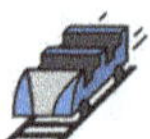 ## JOURNAL PROMPT

Think about a time when someone you care about just refused to listen to your opinion or hear your perspective. How did they act toward you? What did they do to let you know that they didn't want to hear what you were saying? Did you try to reason with them? Did it work? Just reflect here on the situation itself and how it felt to be in that position at that moment.

[Note: The goal here is to lean into the experience of what it's like when you feel dismissed or disregarded. I want you to gain insight into how people with ODD feel all the time, whether people intentionally make them feel dismissed or not. This is what people with ODD carry into the world, and we want to cultivate some insight and empathy for those feelings.]

I'm Emotionally Dysregulated—How Do I Help Myself?

Sometimes your emotions hit so fast and hard, it's like someone slammed a fist on the volume knob and everything's blaring at once. You might feel rage in your chest, shame in your gut, or a flood of tears you didn't see coming. Maybe your hands shake, your heart pounds, and words start flying before you even know what you're saying.

That's emotional dysregulation—when your inner world feels chaotic and charged, limiting your ability to pause, think, reason or respond in a thoughtful way. Basically, this state of being creates intense, prolonged reactions that you may find really hard to recover from.

When you are in this state, the outside world might label you as difficult, dramatic or "a chaos monster," but emotional dysregulation is not really something that one actively chooses. Instead, it's our body, mind, and spirit's way of processing difficult emotions when we haven't been taught how to do so, or when we've experienced trauma or even because of our genetic makeup.

If you're emotionally dysregulated, you can start by asking yourself a key question: *Am I OK with letting my emotions always take the lead?*

If you're reading this, you're probably not.

Then ask: *Am I open to trying one or two things to help me work with my emotions? Am I OK using my emotions as a guide to help me stay steady, instead of viewing them as a dictator controlling my every decision and move?*

This can often be a hard question, because no one may have ever asked us to take stock of our emotions, our triggers, and our overall mental health—so if you're hesitant, it makes total sense. This isn't about being perfect. It's about learning how to stay present, identify your emotions, and work with them, because they really do serve a purpose; they teach you things constantly, and it's important to make sure that you control the volume and never allow them to get so loud that they drown out your ability to think, plan, and execute on your terms.

Let's get into some techniques that can help you come back to yourself—without pretending you're fine, and without letting everything spiral.

1. **Come back to a neutral heart space.** This isn't about forcing yourself to "feel nothing." It's about finding the middle ground between total shutdown and total explosion. Try placing your hand on your chest and breathing into that space—slowly, gently. Imagine your heart softening. Even a few deep breaths here can shift the intensity.

2. **Use grounding techniques from yoga or meditation.** These aren't just for people who sit cross-legged on mountaintops. Try this: feel your feet on the floor. Notice five things you can see, four you can touch, three you can hear, two you can smell, and one you can taste. This gets you back into your body and out of the storm.

3. **Try box breathing.** This one's easy: Breathe in for four counts, hold for four, exhale for four, hold for four. Repeat a few times. It gives your nervous system a reset—like hitting pause on a video before it spirals out of control.

4. **Walk away if you need to.** Yes, *you* can walk away. Anyone can. Walking away doesn't mean you're weak—it means you're wise enough to know that staying might push things further than you want. You can still be angry and compassionate. You can hold your fire *without* letting it burn the room down.

5. **Let your phone be your ally, not your trap.** Instead of doomscrolling or rage-posting, text someone you trust. The one who knows how to help you level out. The one who won't fuel the drama but will help you find your calm. You don't have to go through this alone.

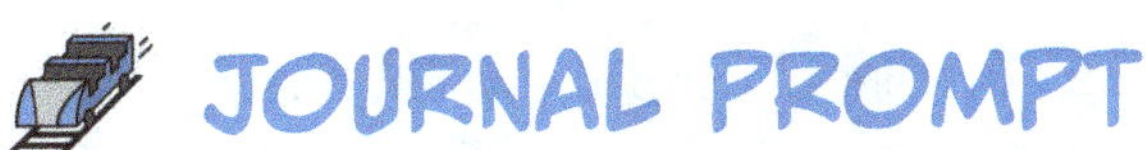

JOURNAL PROMPT

Which of the suggestions for helping yourself lit you up the most? Why? In what ways can you start incorporating them into your life to help you find and keep your center?

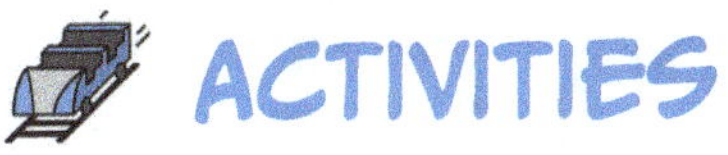

ACTIVITIES

Now that you know something about how to handle emotional dysregulation, even when it's really intense, let's practice some new skills.

EASY

Finding Your Neutral Heart Space

Sometimes, everything inside feels loud—like your thoughts, your feelings, your reactions are all turned up to full volume. When that happens, it can help to find your way back to something quieter. Something steadier. A neutral heart space.

Start by sitting somewhere comfortable—your bed, a chair, even the floor. Close your eyes if that feels OK, and take a few slow breaths. In through your nose, out through your mouth. Let your shoulders drop. Let your belly soften.

Now think about what's been feeling loud lately. Maybe it's someone who upset you, something that didn't go your way, or a situation that's just been hard. Without judging it, just notice it. Give it a name in your mind. Then imagine gently setting it beside you—not ignoring it, just not holding it so tight for now.

Bring your attention to the center of your chest. That space over your heart. Ask yourself: *What does calm feel like in me?* Not happiness. Not sadness. Just calm. Even if it's the tiniest bit—like one small patch of blue sky on a cloudy day—let yourself notice it.

Stay with that feeling for a few breaths. Let it be enough.

When you're ready, open your eyes. You've just found your way back to the middle zone—the part of you that isn't pulled in every direction. From here, you can choose what to do next, not because you're trying to win or prove anything, but because you've come home to yourself.

After this activity, I feel:

MODERATE

Rock of Peace and Power

Let's say you're outside—maybe in your backyard, on the sidewalk, in the park, or just wandering after school—and something catches your eye: a small rock. It doesn't have to be fancy. Just one that feels right in your hand. Maybe it's smooth and cool, maybe it's a little rough around the edges—kind of like a mood, honestly.

Next time you see a rock like that, I want you to pick it up. This rock is going to be your secret reminder, your anchor. Slip it into your backpack, your purse, your sports bag, even your jacket pocket—whatever you carry with you most often. For the next week, that rock travels with you.

Every time something starts to get under your skin—whether it's a friend ghosting you, a text that makes your stomach twist, or a feeling that doesn't even have a name—reach for the rock. Hold it. Feel its weight. And say quietly (or in your head if you're around people): "In this moment, I reclaim my peace."

Then pause. Take four deep, slow breaths. With each one, picture yourself settling—like a snow globe after you shake it. The storm swirls, then calms. Remind yourself: *I am capable. I can handle this. Even if this feeling is big, I don't have to drown in it.*

But that's not all. At some point during the day—maybe after you brush your teeth or just before bed—check in with yourself. How are you feeling? Give it a number from 1 to 10, where 1 is totally wrecked and 10 is flying high. But don't stop at the number. Write down a few words about what's happening: what made you laugh, what felt heavy, what was just OK.

Start noticing patterns. What lifts you up? What tends to knock you down? And just as important—what kind of moments feel like neither? The ordinary, neutral ones. The ones where you're just breathing, just being. That place—not sky-high, not buried low—is actually your inner home. That's the space to return to when the emotional waves start pulling at your feet.

This exercise will help you notice that you have power—even in the smallest ways—to shift your day, your mood, your story. And it all starts with a rock in your pocket.

After this activity, I feel:

HARD

Pausing for Kindness

Here's something gentle to try—something that might feel small at first but can quietly shift the way your whole day unfolds. For the next two weeks, give yourself just five minutes every morning. Before your phone. Before school. Before the scroll. Sit up in bed or on the floor or wherever feels calm. Let your eyes rest on one spot, or close them altogether. You don't need incense or a meditation cushion or anything fancy—just you, breathing.

Now begin to whisper to yourself, slowly: "I forgive myself for riding the wave of negative automatic thinking."

Say it again. And again. Let the words move through you. You don't have to force them to feel true—just offer them. You don't even have to push away the hard thoughts. All you need to do is recognize that they come and go like waves, and forgive yourself for getting swept up in them sometimes. That's human.

Stay with this for five minutes. Not with the aim of fixing anything, but simply to sit with yourself. And when those five minutes end, try something most people forget to do: Carry the calm with you.

Over the course of your day, take tiny pauses. Just a minute here and there—between classes, walking to practice, brushing your teeth, waiting for the bus. No one even has to know you're doing it. Five times a day is enough. When you do, say to yourself: "I remember to extend grace to myself first."

Let it be like a hand on your own shoulder. A gentle voice that says: "You're doing your best. And even when you're not, you still deserve kindness."

These aren't magic spells. But if you keep at them, they start to grow roots inside you. They change the tone of your thoughts. And one day, maybe without realizing it, you'll respond to your own inner storms not with shame, but with softness.

After this activity, I feel:

KEY TAKEAWAYS

Congrats! You made it to the end of Mindset 4: Ride the Roller Coaster! Have you learned anything you want to incorporate into your daily routine? Is there anything in this section you want to shout from the rooftops about? Maybe you've learned something you can share with your friends or parents/caregivers to help them. Make a note of your key takeaways (including the ones you'd like to share with others) and write them below:

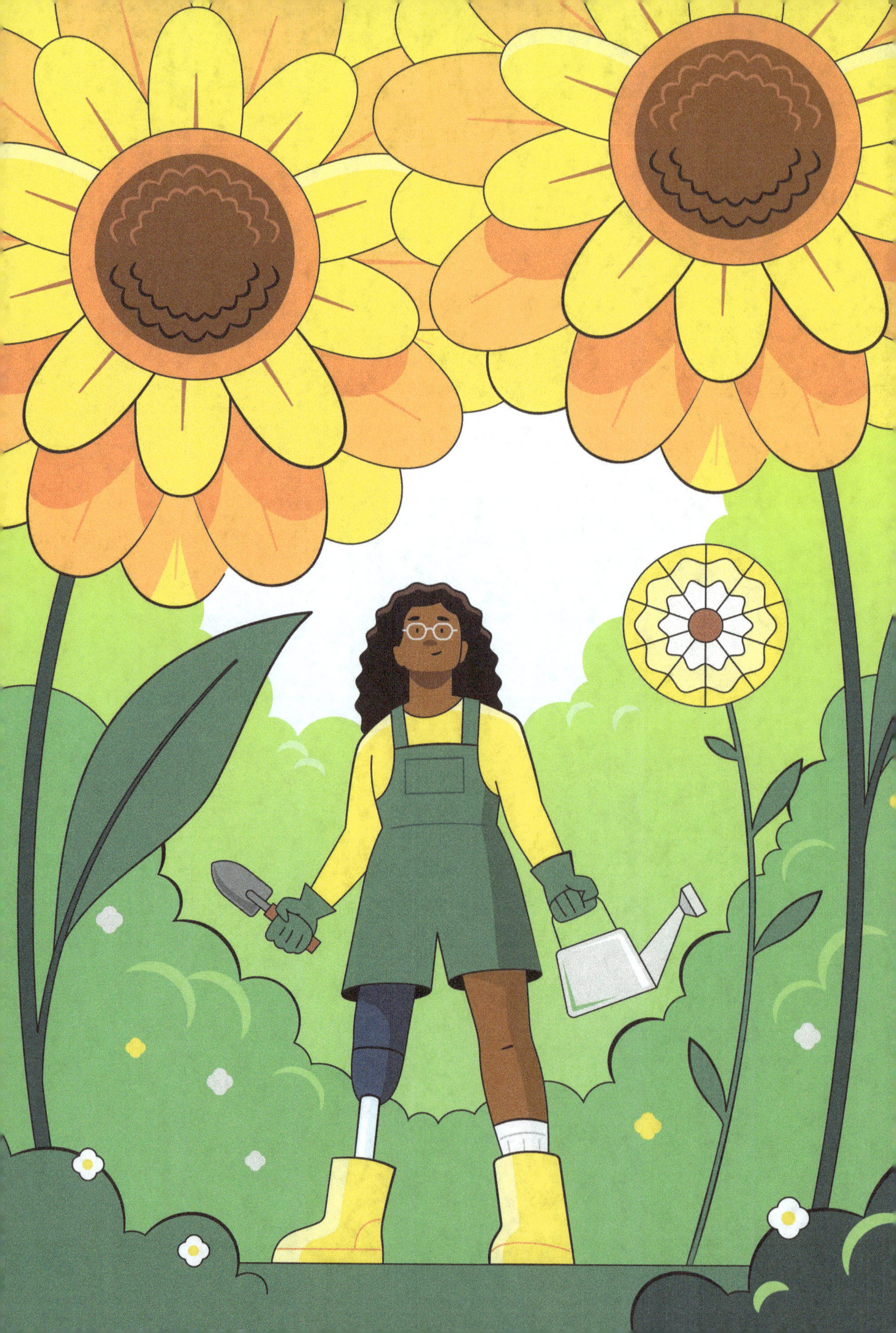

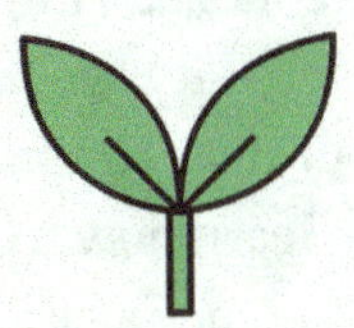

Tend Your Stress, Nurture Your Growth

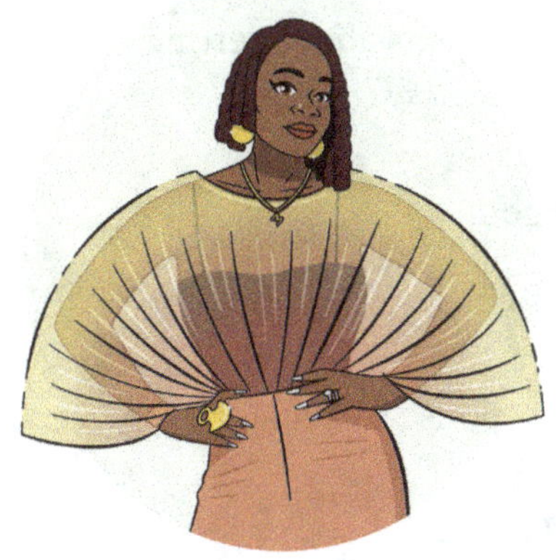

Managing stress isn't just about calming down—it's about *leveling up*. Think of your emotions like video-game characters. When life throws challenges your way—school drama, family stuff, anxiety, trauma triggers—hopefully the right character shows up to help you navigate the challenge or level. And, plot twist: The stressors aren't the enemy sent to destroy you. They're the boosters that help you learn and flex new skills.

Every time you pause to take a deep breath instead of snapping back, or choose to talk it out instead of shutting down, you're unlocking a new level. It might not feel epic in the moment, but that's growth in action. Stress and growth are part of the same quest. You don't get stronger by avoiding the hard levels—you get stronger by learning how to move through them with more awareness and less panic. Every time you walk through a stressful situation, you grab that booster and move up to the next level of emotional intelligence.

Now, let's talk about trauma for a sec. Exposure to traumatic events can make stress responses go haywire: You might freeze, your heart might race, you might feel like shutting down. And while it doesn't feel good, all of this is your body's way of protecting you.

When we are exposed to trauma, our bodies are simply telling us that we've encountered something that feels overwhelming and that has an outsized impact on our bodies, minds, and spirits. Since the dawn of humanity, we have needed something called a fight-or-flight response for our own safety. Trauma exposure leans into that response, and it's up to us to learn how to manage it.

Once again (and I'll keep reminding you), none of this is about getting it "perfect." It's about recognizing patterns and learning how to steady yourself when the situation feels like too much.

By the end of this section, you will know more about:

- Eustress and distress—what they are and the challenges and opportunities associated with them
- Adjustment disorder and how this can be a response to a major stressful life event
- Trauma and post-traumatic stress disorder (PTSD)
- Grief
- Healthy coping skills for grief and trauma
- Post-traumatic growth and the ways our authenticity can emerge from our pain

Let's Get Started

Imagine waking up every day and going to a job where nobody really trusts each other, people are always low-key (or high-key) arguing, the vibe is just off, and no one tells you that you're doing a good job. On top of that, you're the only Black woman or Woman of Color in a leadership role in the entire place—which can feel like carrying the weight of a whole community on your shoulders while no one around you really sees you. That was my life when I first became a psychiatry professor.

I was working full time, leading a team, juggling way too many responsibilities, and then—my spouse and I added two beautiful babies into the mix. I love my babies deeply, and was happy to care for my little muffins, but some days, given the enormous stress of that job, I honestly felt like I was falling apart. I'd sit in my car before walking into work, heart pounding, wishing I didn't have to deal with the foolishness I would most certainly encounter once inside. I was made to feel invisible. I was frustrated. Sad. Stressed with a capital S.

Then—bam—my mom, my best friend, got sick. Really sick. And there was not much we could do to help her but ease her pain. All of this weighed on me. HEAVILY. And eventually, I realized I couldn't keep using myself up just trying to function. I needed help. So I found a psychologist—Dr. M— who helped me name what I was dealing with: racism, sexism, burnout, and the kind of pressure that makes you question your worth. And she told me something I'll never forget: "None of this is your fault. But you *do* deserve tools to cope until you're in a better place."

That's when she introduced me to *mindfulness meditation*. She told me about a book (*Wherever You Go, There You Are* by Dr. Jon Kabat-Zinn) and gave me a guided meditation CD. Yep, this was way before Spotify playlists and Calm app notifications.

At first, I honestly didn't know what to make of all of it. Then I *really* tried it—sitting still, breathing, tuning in instead of fighting through—it was like finding a little island of calm in the middle of a storm. I made a decision: Every morning, before the sun was even up, I got out of bed at 4:30 a.m. I'd meditate for thirty to sixty minutes. *Every day.* Then I'd get my kids ready, get myself together, and head into work.

Meditation became my armor. My daily vaccine against stress. It didn't fix the system I was stuck in, but it helped me stay grounded, connected to myself, and less reactive when things got rough. For ten years, I used that morning practice to survive a really hard chapter of my life—until I was finally able to move on and create a job that respected me (the job I created as founder and president of The AAKOMA Project).

If you're dealing with chaos—at school, at home, online—please remember that meditation really is for anyone and everyone trying to stay sane in a world that sometimes makes you feel like you're drowning. Even just five minutes a day can help you come back to *you*. And you know what I'm gonna tell you—you're ALWAYS worth coming back to.

 ## What Is Stress?

Let's break down stress in a way that actually makes sense—because we all feel it, but nobody really sits us down and explains what's going on inside our bodies and minds when life gets *a lot*.

Here's the official definition from the American Psychological Association (fancy, right?): "the physiological or psychological response to internal or external stressors."[12] Let's put it another way: Stress is the way your

---

12. American Psychological Association. "Definition of Stress." American Psychological Association, n.d. https://www.apa.org/topics/stress.

body and mind react to stuff that throws you off balance—things happening *outside* you, like a fight with a friend or too many deadlines, or *inside* you, like self-doubt or overthinking.

Most of the time when people say they're "stressed out," they mean they're dealing with **distress**—the not-so-fun kind of stress. This is the heavy feeling that makes your stomach twist, your heart race, or your brain feel foggy and overwhelmed. It can show up when you're cramming for a test, worrying about your future, or feeling like no one gets you.

But did you know there's also a good kind of stress? It's called **eustress** (yōō-stress). Sounds weird, but it's legit. Eustress is the type of stress that actually helps you. It's that little nudge that pushes you to do something important—like getting off TikTok to finally stretch your tired eyes, or standing up to give a speech even though you're nervous, because deep down, you care. It's like your inner coach saying, "This matters. Let's do it."

Now, why does stress matter so much, especially when it comes to you?

Because research has shown that young people today—*you*—are carrying more stress than past generations. Not just school stress, but social pressures, climate anxiety, family stuff, identity struggles, and a world that can feel straight-up exhausting. And for people in marginalized communities, there's often another layer of stress—navigating racism, sexism, homophobia, classism . . . things that don't always get named, but are deeply felt.

Stress doesn't show up the same way for everyone. For some, it looks like snapping at people. For others, it's zoning out, feeling tired all the time, or constantly doubting yourself. That's why it's so important to know your own signals—and to learn how to cope in ways that don't hurt you or shut you down. You deserve to feel empowered—not buried.

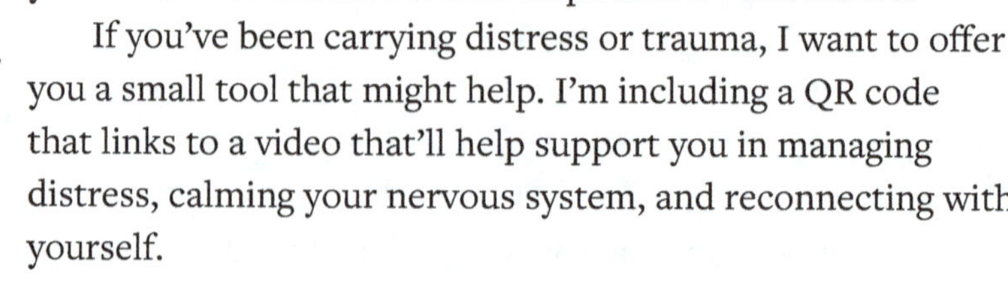

If you've been carrying distress or trauma, I want to offer you a small tool that might help. I'm including a QR code that links to a video that'll help support you in managing distress, calming your nervous system, and reconnecting with yourself.

 JOURNAL PROMPT

When you think about stress in your own life, what does it feel like? Where do you notice it—in your body, your headspace, your habits? Try to recall a time when you felt really overwhelmed. What was happening? How did it feel in your body? Where did you feel it (your stomach, your throat, your head, etc.)? What was the trigger (i.e., what thing started the spiral into stress)? Now think about how you responded. Did you shut down, zone out, push through, get irritable, or try to keep it all together for everyone else? What helped you get through it? What didn't help the situation at all?

This is a space to be curious and honest with yourself—no judgment, just learning to understand your own stress story.

Signs and Symptoms of Stress

Let's check in on how you've been feeling lately—like, <u>really</u> feeling. Over the past week or two, have you noticed signs that stress might be building up? Stress isn't always a bad thing, but when it piles on or goes unrecognized, it can mess with your energy, focus, and mood.

Here are some common signs of everyday stress that might be showing up in your life:

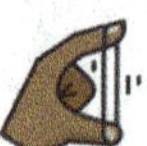 Feeling tense, overwhelmed, or like your brain is in five places at once

 Clenching your jaw or fists without realizing it

 Procrastinating even on stuff you usually enjoy (school, hobbies, plans with friends)

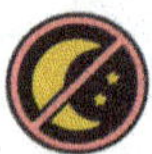 Trouble sleeping because your mind won't shut off

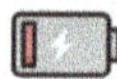 Feeling constantly tired—even if you slept enough

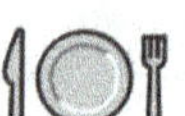 Reaching for comfort food (or skipping meals without meaning to)

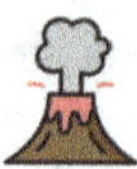 Snapping at people or getting annoyed way faster than usual

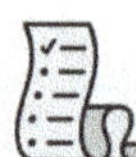 Feeling stuck in a loop of "I have so much to do and no time/energy to do it"

But not all stress is bad. Remember, there's also eustress—the kind that gets your heart racing in a <u>good</u> way:

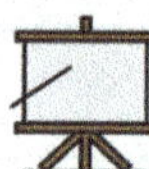 Giving a class presentation or performing in front of others

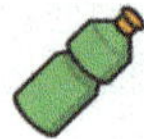 Preparing for a big game or competition

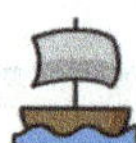 Pushing yourself to try something new or challenging

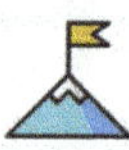 Working toward a goal that actually matters to you

 Your heart flutters and you feel butterflies

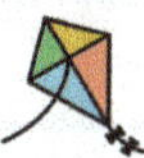 You feel a lightness inside you, like you're floating on air

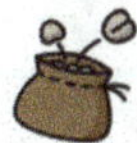 You feel antsy (can't sit still) with anticipation

Eustress helps you grow—it means you care, you're stretching, you're alive. But if too much stress (even the "good" kind) stacks up without enough recovery time, your system can still crash.

The key is noticing your signals and triggers. What's your stress coping style? What helps you come back to center (that neutral heart space we talked about in Mindset 4)? Keep reading to learn how to work with your stress instead of letting it run the show.

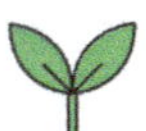 JOURNAL PROMPT

Think about a time when you felt pushed in a good way—like you were challenged, but it made you feel alive or motivated. Maybe it was performing, competing, speaking up, trying something new, or working toward a goal that mattered to you. What did that kind of good stress feel like in your body? How did it affect your focus, energy, or confidence?

Now think about a time when the pressure became too much. Maybe your heart was racing, or you felt frozen, foggy, or exhausted. Maybe even the stuff you usually like started to feel overwhelming. What changed? Was there a moment when the stress tipped from helpful to heavy?

The goal isn't to avoid stress altogether, but to understand your signals. What does it feel like when you're in your growth zone, and what does it feel like when you've crossed into overload? What helps you come back to balance when you've gone too far? Start to notice where that edge lives for you—and what you need when you get close to it.

When Change Is Too Big to Face Alone

Alright, let's talk about something that doesn't get talked about enough—but should: **adjustment disorder**.

You're going through a big change—maybe a breakup, switching schools, your parents separating, losing a friendship, or even something that seems small to others but feels *huge* to you. Normally, yeah, of course that would be stressful. But sometimes, the stress doesn't fade. It lingers. It messes with your head. You can't concentrate, you feel overwhelmed, your emotions are all over the place—and everything that used to feel doable suddenly feels impossible.

That's what adjustment disorder can feel like. It's like stress on overdrive. You're not just reacting to a tough situation—you're stuck in it, emotionally. It hits hard, and it can be paralyzing.

Adjustment disorder is a real mental health condition. It's short term, but that doesn't mean it's not serious. A lot of people go through it at some point in their lives—especially when change hits fast and hard.

Some signs that you might be dealing with adjustment disorder include:

- Feeling down or hopeless
- Lots of worry or anxiety
- Not sleeping well
- Trouble focusing (like, even TikToks feel like too much)
- Getting angry fast or acting out
- Feeling stuck, alone, or like you've lost confidence in yourself

The key thing mental-health professionals look for is this: Are your emotional reactions way bigger or more intense than what's expected for the situation? And are those feelings seriously messing with your life—school, friendships, family, your overall vibe? If yes, it might be adjustment disorder.

It usually shows up within three months of a stressful event. And nope—it's not the same as grief, which we'll get into in a bit. If someone is grieving the loss of a person or pet or something deeply meaningful, that's a different process.

But when it's adjustment disorder, there are different types—like:

- With depressed mood
- With anxiety
- With both depressed and anxious mood
- With behavioral changes (like acting out, getting into fights, skipping class)

The good news is, it's totally *treatable*. Therapy can help a ton—especially if you talk to someone who listens without judgment. And sometimes, even just naming what's going on—saying, "Hey, this *isn't* just me being dramatic or lazy"—is the first step toward healing. So if change has knocked you flat, and you feel like you've lost your way, take a breath. You're not broken. You're reacting to something real—and there *are* ways to move through it.

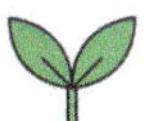 # JOURNAL PROMPT

Think about a time when you experienced a really big change. Maybe you had to move away from your friends and family. Maybe you failed a class and were faced with retaking it. Maybe the dream job turned out to be a nightmare. What did it feel like when you realized the change was happening or needed to happen? What emotions did you experience? Where did you feel those emotions in your body? Take a moment to reflect on the overall experience—this can give you some insight into how you cope with stress and what types of situations trigger stress for you.

The Truth About Trauma

You've probably heard the words *trauma* and *PTSD* thrown around all the time lately. People say things like, "Ugh, I'm so traumatized by that test," or "That movie gave me PTSD." But do we actually understand what those words mean?

Let's break it down together.

According to the American Psychological Association (yep, the professionals who study the mind), **psychological trauma** is an intense emotional response that "involves events that pose significant threat (physical, emotional, or psychological) to the safety of the victim or loved ones/ friends and are overwhelming and shocking."[13] This could be something like experiencing or witnessing violence, losing someone you love, or living through a natural disaster.

Then there's **PTSD**, which stands for **Post-Traumatic Stress Disorder**, defined as occurring "when someone lives through or witnesses an event in which they believe that there is a threat to life or physical integrity and safety and experiences fear, terror, or helplessness."[14]

In both trauma and PTSD, there's something intense that happens. It hits hard emotionally. And for people from marginalized communities— Those with disabilities, People of Color, LGBTQAI+ folks, immigrants— there's another layer: the trauma tied to identity. We're talking racism,

---

13. American Psychological Association. "Definition of Trauma." American Psychological Association, n.d. https://www.apa.org/topics/trauma.
14. American Psychological Association. "Definition of PTSD." American Psychological Association, n.d. https://www.apa.org/topics/ptsd.

homophobia, transphobia, xenophobia, and more. These aren't just "bad experiences." They're often everyday realities, especially in this day and age. And it's not something anyone chooses or can control.

This is why it's so important to normalize conversations about trauma and PTSD. We live in a world where so much is happening all the time—and we're constantly seeing it on our phones, in the news, in our feeds. From climate disasters to political chaos to economic stress, we're surrounded by what some experts call **collective trauma**—trauma that affects whole communities or even the world.

However, sometimes people casually use words like *trauma* or *toxic* when they really just mean "that was annoying" or "we disagreed." And while it's great that mental health is being talked about more, it's also important to understand two key things about real trauma:

1. Trauma is personal. What deeply affects one person might not faze another at all. There's no one-size-fits-all when it comes to emotional pain.
2. You don't have to *live through* something to be traumatized by it. That's where vicarious trauma comes in.

Vicarious trauma is when someone is affected by hearing about or witnessing another person's traumatic experience. This happens a lot with therapists, doctors, and social workers—they sit with people during their hardest moments, and over time, that can take a serious emotional toll. But it also happens to young people like you, especially now.

In research on the mental health of young People of Color (that's you and your peers), 34% said they had experienced racial trauma often or very often in their lives. Further, across all racial ethnic groups, close to half of Latino/é youth and young adults report racial trauma experiences (44.6%). And when it comes to vicarious racial trauma, young people said they felt it most through social media (32.4%) and the news (25.9%).[15] Think about it—when your feed is filled with stories of people who look like you being hurt, silenced, or mistreated, it sticks with you.

Another form of trauma that's rarely talked about—but very real—is **intergenerational trauma**. This is the emotional pain passed down from parents, grandparents, and great-grandparents. Maybe it came from surviving colonization, war, slavery, forced migration, cultural erasure, or other heinous and violent acts of injustice and dehumanization. Maybe

---

15. Breland-Noble, A., The AAKOMA Project, and C. A. Harb. *State of Mental Health of Youth and Young Adults of Color,* Full Report. 2025.

your family never talked about it directly, but you *felt* it. Maybe they did talk about it—and it stayed with you. Even if they didn't mean to, they might have passed down a kind of anxiety or fear that they were never able to work through themselves.

That's why I try to give older adults grace—loving patience. A lot of them were never given the space or support to heal. They were told to just survive, to push through, to act like emotional pain didn't matter. Some even believed that talking about your feelings was a "luxury" or "first-world problem." But you? You have something powerful.

You have the emotional freedom to heal.

You don't have to carry all that pain alone. And you don't have to wait for permission. You already have it. When you prioritize your healing— through therapy, through rest, through creativity, through community— you're not just helping yourself. You're showing the people around you that healing is possible for them, too. Even the ones who never thought they deserved it.

And that's what I want for you. Not just to get by. Not just to cope. I want you to *thrive*. To feel free. To feel seen. To feel whole. And I want you to know—you have full permission to heal.

To learn more about the different forms of trauma, check out the video linked in the QR code here.

Grief Is How We Heal

Let's take a minute to talk about grief. Yeah, that tricky, unpredictable emotion that shows up like an uninvited guest and refuses to leave when we want it to.

Grief is what we feel when we've lost something or someone important to us. It's not just for death—though that's definitely a big one. We grieve for all kinds of things: leaving middle school for high school, losing a friendship, moving away, getting tough news about our health, or even saying goodbye to who we used to be.

Bottom line is, grieving is healthy. It's your mind and body reacting to an experience that's hard or painful. When we don't acknowledge it, grief doesn't disappear—it just finds other ways to show up. And it's not the same for everyone. There's no one-size-fits-all timeline or "right" way to do it.

I remember feeling a wave of sadness and panic at the end of my time at Howard University. Graduation should've felt like a win, but I was scared. I was leaving behind a familiar world and moving to New York—no friends, no family, no idea what came next. Back then, I thought I was just being anxious. Now I understand: I was grieving. I was mourning a version of my life that was ending, and that feeling was real and totally valid.

Grief isn't linear. There's no neat beginning, middle, and end. Some days you'll feel OK, and then suddenly something—a smell, a song, a memory—can hit you out of nowhere. That's not weakness. That's being human.

And grief isn't just emotional—it's physical, too. Some people sleep too much or not at all. Some get headaches, stomachaches, or back pain. Others lose or gain a lot of weight. Our bodies carry our sadness even when our minds don't know what to do with it.

There's also a big cultural piece to grief. In the U.S., a lot of people treat grief like a short-term thing you just "get over." You get a few sick days off and then you're expected to bounce back. But in many cultures around the world, grief is sacred. It's a process. A rite of passage.

I interviewed Dr. Helen Hsu, a mental health expert in the AAPI community, on my podcast *Couched in Color*. She told me about her Vietnamese American coworker who wore a black armband for a year after his mother died. Everyone at the office knew what it meant—and they treated him with extra respect and compassion. That's a powerful way of saying, "I'm grieving, please see me."

Another example? In many Latino communities, there's Día de los Muertos, the Day of the Dead. It's more than an opportunity to mourn those loved ones who've passed—it's about celebrating their lives. It gives people space to feel their sadness *and* their love at the same time.

These traditions teach us something essential: Grief isn't something to fear. It's part of what it means to be alive and to care deeply.

And yet, so many of us don't know how to ask for help when we're grieving. We don't know what to say to someone who's hurting. That's fine—we're all learning. But what matters is that we *try*.

Here's one thing you can do: Just be a witness. You don't have to fix someone's pain, or say the perfect thing. You just have to show up. Sit with them. Be there. And don't make it about you. You can say something like: "I've been through loss, but this isn't about me. I'm here for you, in whatever way you need."

Or you can ask: "Is there something I can do for you right now? Even if the answer is no, I'm still here."

Grief deserves our attention. It deserves our patience. And weird as it sounds, grief is a kind of love. It's how we honor what mattered to us. That's why it's also OK to laugh, to dance, to celebrate even as we grieve. We're really meant to hold space for all of it: the sadness, the love, the memories, and the joy that can surprise us in the midst of it all.

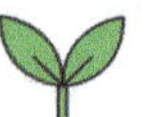 JOURNAL PROMPT

Look around at the world today—how do you see grief showing up in the people and communities around you, especially the ones you're a part of? What losses—personal, collective, cultural—seem to be weighing on them?

Have you ever felt someone else's grief seep into your own heartspace? What was that like? How did it affect the way you moved through your days, or how you saw your own pain?

Now turn inward: When you've faced grief—whether from losing someone, something, or some version of yourself—what helped you carry it? What didn't? What made the weight heavier, and what, even briefly, helped you breathe?

If grief is a kind of terrain we're all destined to cross, what are the handholds, the resting places, the small signs of life that remind you it's OK to keep going?

I've Experienced Trauma—How Do I Help Myself?

You've probably noticed that people talk about trauma *a lot* these days. It's on the news, all over social media, YouTube, even in school and at work. And with all that talk, it can sometimes feel like you're the only one who doesn't fully get what trauma is—or how to handle it. If that's you, don't worry. You're not alone, and there *is* a way to understand and deal with it.

But first, you've got to learn how to recognize and name your emotions. That way, you don't end up getting dragged around by what other people think or feel, like a tree blowing wildly in the wind. The more you know what's going on inside you, the more grounded you'll be.

Second, you've got to learn how to reach out when you're going through something hard. That includes the moments right after trauma, which can be especially tough because trauma often makes people want to pull away and shut down. This is called **dissociation**, and it's one way the brain tries to protect us. But if we let ourselves completely disconnect, we can end up feeling even more isolated—which makes healing harder.

So instead of shutting down, we want to practice something called **interdependence**. That means finding a healthy balance: protecting the parts of yourself that need space while also letting people in and asking for help when you need it. It's not all or nothing—it's about creating connection *and* boundaries.

Now, let's talk about a specific type of trauma that doesn't get talked about enough: **identity-based trauma**. This includes things like:

- Racial trauma (caused by racism or discrimination)
- Homophobia and transphobia
- Ableism (discrimination against people with disabilities)

- Xenophobia (fear or hatred of immigrants or people from other countries)
- Islamophobia, and other kinds of prejudice

These kinds of trauma aren't experienced by everyone, but they seriously impact people in marginalized communities. And for way too long, People of Color and others with intersecting identities have been told to stay quiet about it. To ignore it. To blend in without making a fuss. That silence? That pressure to "just deal"? It adds to the trauma.

In this book, we're not doing that. We're saying the truth out loud. Naming your trauma—especially identity-based trauma—is one way to erase shame and blame. It helps us take back our power.

Here's some data to show what this looks like for young people today.

IN THE 2025 SOMHYOC REPORT[16]:

- **34%** of Youth and Young Adults of Color (YYAC) said they experience racial trauma often or very often.
- The top sources of trauma for YYAC are:
    - Social media (**32.4%**)
    - Police (**26.5%**)
    - The news (**25.9%**)

FOR QUEER YOUTH:

- **44.6%** of LGBTQAI+ YYAC said they've had negative comments made about their sexual orientation online.
- About **1 in 3** said they've been bullied online about their physical abilities.

So yes—young people from all kinds of backgrounds *are* facing trauma. That's real.

But here's the hopeful part: something called **post-traumatic growth**. What is that? It's a term coined by psychologists Dr. Richard Tedeschi and Dr. Lawrence Calhoun back in the 1990s. Their research showed that even though trauma is painful, it can also be the start of real personal growth.

---

16. Breland-Noble, A., The AAKOMA Project, and C. A. Harb. *State of Mental Health of Youth and Young Adults of Color,* Full Report. 2025.

According to their theory: "People who endure psychological struggle following adversity can often see positive growth afterward."[17]

In other words, trauma can be the beginning of something powerful. If we face it—really work through it—it can actually help us grow stronger, more compassionate, and more connected to ourselves and others. But that growth doesn't happen by accident. It takes conscious effort and action.

So what can you do to move toward healing and growth after trauma? That's where we're headed next—looking at real, tangible steps you can take to manage extreme stress and begin your healing journey.

1. **Name the trauma.** Can you describe what happened to you—and how it made you feel? If not, that's OK. This is the best place to begin. Being able to name your trauma is powerful. It helps you understand the root of your pain, which makes it easier to focus on what kind of healing you actually need. Think of it like trying to treat a wound—you have to know *where* it is and *how* it happened in order to take care of it.

2. **Identify the trigger.** Now try to zoom in a little more. What specific part of the experience hurt you the most? Let's say someone experienced intimate partner violence (IPV)—which, sadly, can happen to people as young as twelve or thirteen. That kind of trauma can include both emotional and physical harm. The overall experience might be traumatic, but it's just as important to notice which moments still hit hard when you think about them. What parts make you flinch or feel sick, even years later? Those are your triggers, and the more you understand them, the more you can build ways to cope.

3. **Learn to use your breath.** This one might sound simple, but it's seriously powerful. Your breath is free, it goes everywhere with you, and it can calm your nervous system in moments of stress. Deep breathing helps clear your head, reduce stress, and even lower something called **cortisol**—that's the hormone your body releases when you're under pressure. For People of Color especially, learning how to manage cortisol levels is really important because high cortisol over time can mess with

17. Collier, L. "Growth after Trauma." Monitor on Psychology, November 2016. https://www.apa.org/monitor/2016/11/growth-trauma; Tedeschi, R. G., and L. Calhoun. "Posttraumatic Growth: A New Perspective on Psychotraumatology." Psychiatric Times 21, no. 4 (2004): 58–60.

your body (it can affect your skin, blood pressure, weight, and more). So when things feel overwhelming, try stopping and taking a few slow, deep breaths. It's a small act, but it can shift your entire mood.

4. **Be patient with yourself.** Healing is not a race. It's more like a marathon—or even a long road trip with lots of stops along the way. One thing I used to tell my patients is this: If the trauma lasted a long time, don't expect the healing to happen instantly. That's just not how it works. In our society, people are always saying "just get over it" or "move on"—but that's not how deep healing happens. It takes time, and rushing can actually get in the way. So give yourself some grace. Healing might take months, or even years. That's normal.

5. **Healing is not linear, but it's still happening.** Some days, it might feel like you've taken ten steps forward—and then suddenly, like you've fallen five steps back. That doesn't mean you're failing. It means you're *human*. You might still get triggered by memories years after something happened. But now, you've got tools. You know what your triggers are, you know how to calm yourself down, and you know how to bring yourself back. That's progress. That's growth.

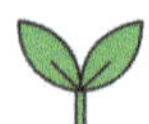 ## JOURNAL PROMPT

Which of the suggestions for helping yourself lit you up the most? Why? Which of these strategies can you start incorporating into your life to help you steady yourself when you feel off balance and to remind you that your pain doesn't make you less than?

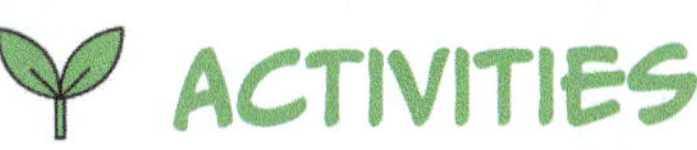 ## ACTIVITIES

Now that you know something about how we can take stressful and trau-matic situations and use them as opportunities for growth, let's practice some new skills.

EASY

Naming Your Stress

Take a moment to name the one thing that's been the most stressful for you over the past two weeks. It could be something obvious, like school or family stuff, or something harder to explain, like feeling overwhelmed or disconnected. Now, for just five minutes, think about the top three reasons this is stressing you out. Ask yourself: *What about this feels hard? Is there something deeper underneath it—like fear, pressure, or feeling stuck?* Don't worry about fixing it right now. Remember Mindset 1? Just naming it is a powerful first step.

After this activity, I feel:

MODERATE

What's Here? What's Missing?

Let's slow things down. Start by taking a few deep breaths—in through your nose, out through your mouth. Let your shoulders drop. Give yourself permission to take this time just for *you*.

Now, over the next thirty minutes, reflect on this: What do you already have within you—or around you—that helps you manage stress, overwhelm, anxiety, or any of the tough stuff we've talked about in this section? These might be actual tools (like journaling, music, breathing, movement), people you trust, or even parts of your own personality—like creativity, humor, or the ability to stay calm.

Then ask yourself: *What's missing?* Is there something you wish you had access to—like a therapist, a quiet space, a creative outlet, or even just more time to rest? Be honest with yourself. What do you think this tool or support could give you? Why would it help?

And finally: Why haven't you used it yet? Maybe you didn't know it existed, or maybe you didn't feel like you were allowed to ask for it. Maybe it felt too far out of reach. There's no judgment here—just curiosity.

MINDSET 5

Use your journal to explore all of this. You're not just listing tools—you're building a map. A map of how you take care of yourself, what's helped you get this far, and what might support you even more moving forward.

After this activity, I feel:

____

____

____

____

____

____

____

HARD

Understanding Trauma

Ever feel like something's going on inside you, but you don't have the words for it? Reading a book about trauma, PTSD, or adjustment disorder can help make sense of what you—or people you care about—might be feeling. It's not just about learning the facts; it's about understanding yourself better and realizing you're not alone. Use the list in the QR code here to find a book that grabs your attention—whether it's a personal story, a guide from a therapist, or something that breaks down the science in a real, relatable way. The more you understand how trauma works, the more power you have to heal, help others, and show up for yourself with compassion.

After this activity, I feel:

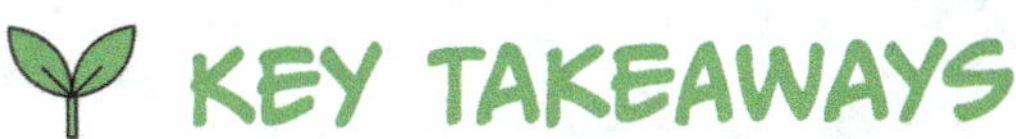 KEY TAKEAWAYS

Congrats! You made it to the end of Mindset 5: Tend Your Stress, Nurture Your Growth! Have you learned anything you want to incorporate into your daily routine? Is there anything in this section you want to shout from the rooftops about? Maybe you've learned something you can share with your friends or parents/caregivers to help them. Make a note of your key takeaways (including the ones you'd like to share with others) and write them below:

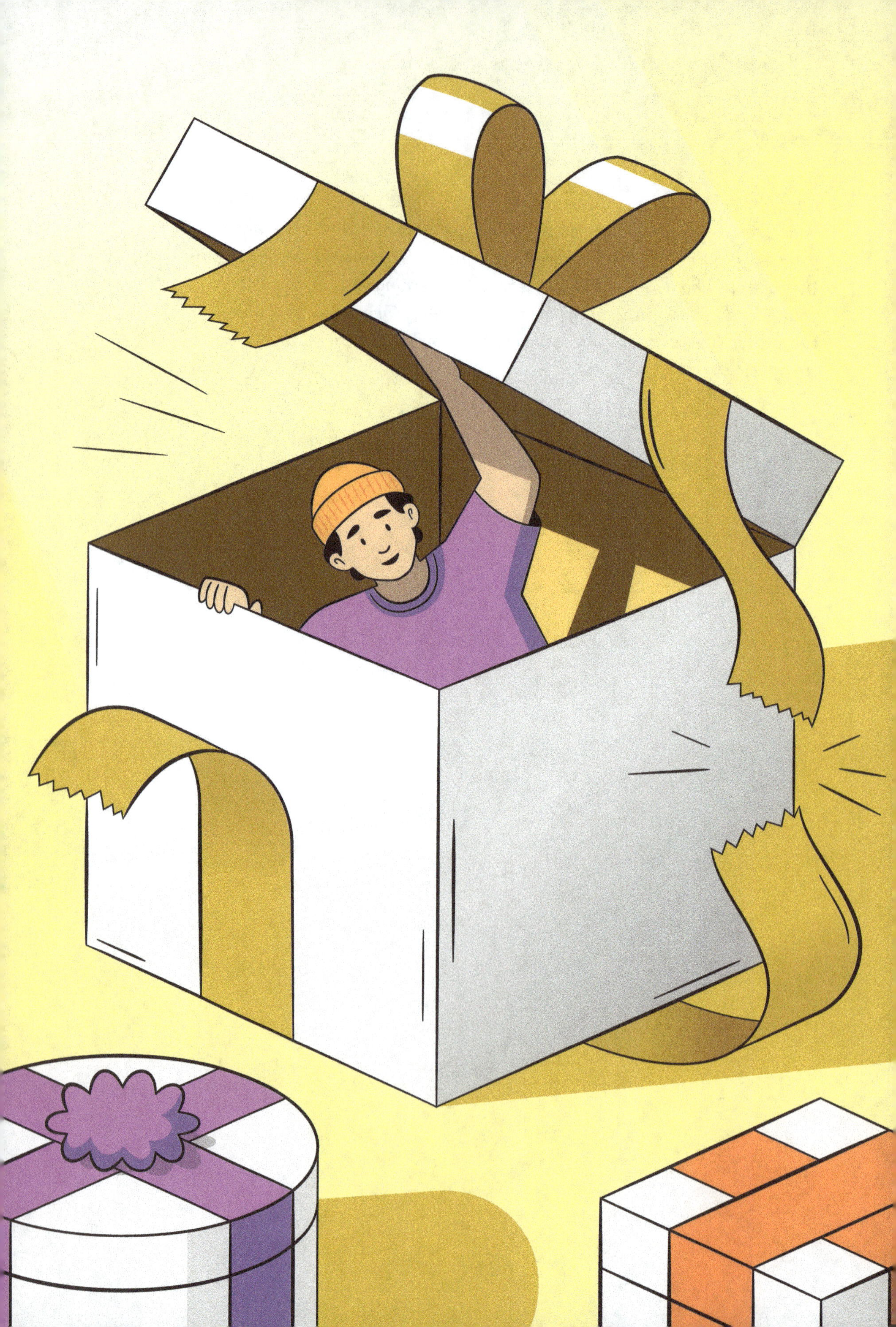

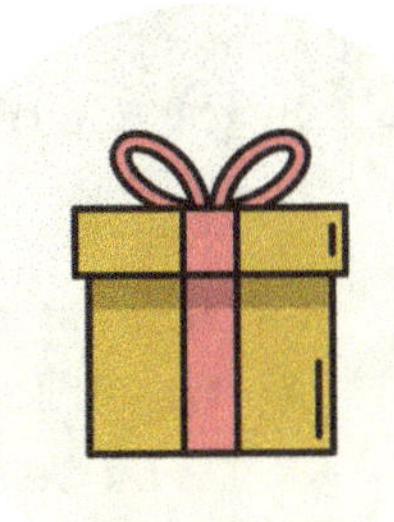

You Are a Gift

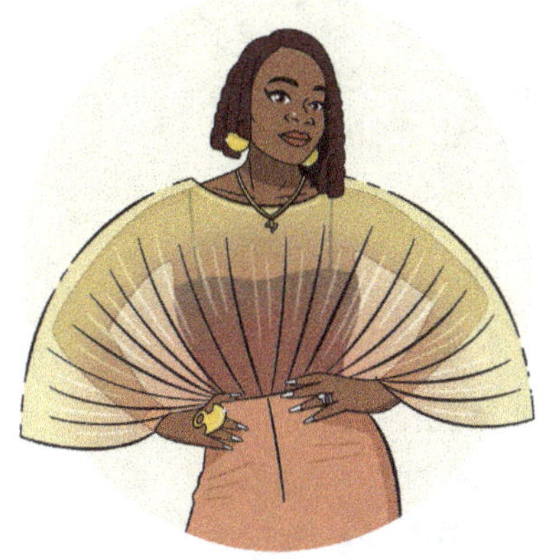

You might not hear this enough, but it's true: *You are a gift.* Full stop. Not when you achieve more, not when you act different, not when you hide the parts of you that feel too big or too messy. Right now. Exactly as you are. You have a light inside you that nobody else can copy, no matter how hard they try. Even if people haven't always seen it—or worse, made you doubt it—your light is real. You are lovable, brilliant, and worthy, just by being you.

Here's a secret most people don't tell you: Self-love isn't something you either "have" or "don't have." It's a skill. Like learning a new language or riding a bike. You practice it. Some days you'll feel strong at it, and other days, it might feel impossible. That's normal. Especially when you've been made to feel alone or unseen. Sometimes, that hurt can sneak in and make you want to turn against yourself, but your pain isn't proof that you're broken. It's proof that you feel deeply, that you care, that you're alive. And those are powerful gifts, too.

Learning to love yourself is about showing up for yourself, even when it's hard. And you don't have to be perfect at it, you just have to keep going. Your story matters. You matter. You always have, and you always will.

By the end of this section, you will know more about:

- Self-love and how to cultivate it
- Self-esteem, self-concept, self-efficacy—and how they all relate to self-love
- Why we sometimes hurt ourselves when we feel we aren't enough (through non-suicidal self-injury and eating disorders)

Let's Get Started

A while back, I worked with a young Man of Color in his early twenties. He was soft-spoken, kind, and honestly just a beautiful soul—but every time we met, he always looked a little sad. He was getting ready to move to a new city for a new job, and while that's supposed to be exciting, he was scared. He had spent years finding friends who *got* him: people who made him feel safe, accepted, and loved for exactly who he was. And now he was terrified he'd have to start all over again. Would he find a circle like that again? Would he be OK?

As we spent more time together, it became clear that a lot of his fears came down to how he felt about himself. He worried about how he looked, how he talked, how he dressed—and deep down, he struggled to believe he was enough. Every time I sat across from him, I could feel how heavy that fear was: the fear of not being accepted, of not trusting yourself to belong anywhere. So many times, I wanted to say to him: "I see such an incredible, amazing human being sitting right in front of me. I wish you could see yourself the way so many of us do." But I didn't, because at the time, that wasn't my role as a mental-health provider.

And here's the thing: I can say that to you, as well. I wish you could see yourself the way so many of us do. You are so much more than your doubts. You are already someone worth loving, exactly as you are. Even if you can't always see your own brilliance right now, please know that the way you see yourself *can* and *will* change over time. It's not set in stone.

Every small act of kindness you show yourself—every time you choose to be in your own corner instead of tearing yourself down—helps build a stronger, more loving relationship with yourself. You don't have to wait for another person to show up for you. You can start showing up for yourself, step by step, choice by choice. You are not your worst days. You are a gift,

MINDSET 6

and learning to stand in solidarity with yourself is one of the most powerful things you will ever do.

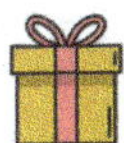 What Does It Mean to Be a Gift?

When I was little, my mom used to tell me, "No one else in this world can love you if you don't first love yourself." I think there's some truth to that, but I also believe it's more complicated. For a lot of us, the first person who's supposed to love us unconditionally is a parent or a caregiver. And when that happens, it can make a huge difference. But the hard truth is, not everyone grows up with someone who knows how to show healthy love. Some parents or caregivers just aren't equipped. And if that's part of your story, I want you to know: *I see you, and I'm so sorry.* You deserve better.

Loving yourself isn't about pretending you're perfect. It's about being able to see the good in yourself even when you mess up or make bad decisions. Self-love doesn't erase the hard stuff life throws at you. But it does teach you that you have what it takes to face it: to admit your mistakes, learn from them, and keep moving forward.

If you come from a marginalized community or a diverse cultural background, you might have been taught different ideas about what it means to "love yourself." And honestly, sometimes those ideas can clash with the dominant culture. In a lot of cultures, the *group*—your family, your community—comes first. Success isn't just about you; it's about what you do for everyone around you. But here in the U.S., the idea of "rugged individualism"—basically, doing it all on your own—is pushed really hard. You can probably feel how those two messages pull in different directions when you think about who you are and what matters most to you.

On top of that, if you have marginalized identities, the media hardly ever shows the full, amazing complexity of who you are. In our *State of Mental Health of Youth and Young Adults of Color 2025* study, almost 30% of AANHPI (Asian American, Native Hawaiian, Pacific Islander) and Arab/MENA (Middle Eastern, North African) youth said there aren't enough influencers who look like them or represent their backgrounds on social media. That's a huge deal. And it's not just social media—the *UCLA Entertainment and Media Research Initiative* reported that in 2023, almost three-quarters of the top streaming movies didn't have even one actor with a known disability in the main cast. In 2025, the numbers barely changed—actually, less than 8% of all on-camera film actors were people with known disabilities.[18]

The truth is, when you don't see people like you reflected in movies, shows, social media, or anywhere else, it can mess with how you see yourself. It can make you feel invisible, like you don't belong. That's why representation matters *so much*. And it's why it can be harder—but also more important—for people with marginalized identities to build strong, loving relationships with ourselves.

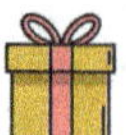 ## JOURNAL PROMPT

If self-love were a person, how would they treat you? What would they say to you when you're proud? What would they say when you're struggling? How would they show up for you, even on the hard days? Take your time. Imagine it clearly. Then ask yourself: How can I start treating myself the way self-love would?

18. https://socialsciences.ucla.edu/initiatives/hollywood-diversity-report/

Signs and Symptoms of Self-Love in Action

You've probably heard the word *self-esteem* before—like when people talk about "having good self-esteem" or "building your self-esteem." But there are a couple other important terms that connect to how we see ourselves, too: *self-concept* and *self-efficacy*. If those words sound unfamiliar, don't worry—you're about to learn what they mean and why they matter.

Spoiler: All three of them—self-esteem, self-concept, and self-efficacy—are huge parts of how we learn to love ourselves.

Let's break it down:

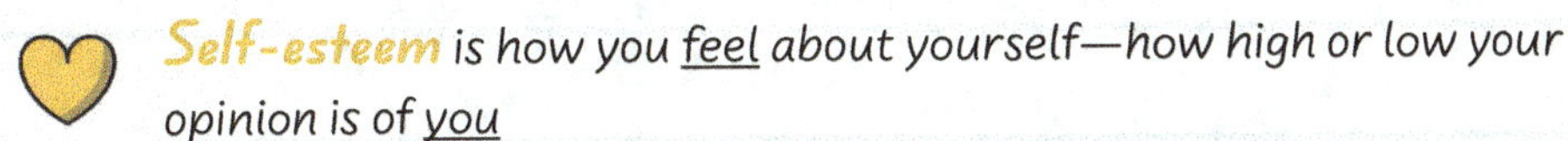 *Self-esteem* is how you <u>feel</u> about yourself—how high or low your opinion is of <u>you</u>

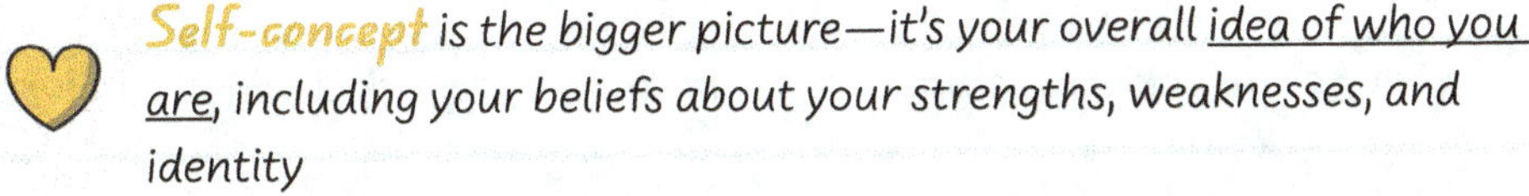 *Self-concept* is the bigger picture—it's your overall <u>idea of who you are</u>, including your beliefs about your strengths, weaknesses, and identity

Self-efficacy is your belief about how good <u>you</u> are at doing things— it's how much <u>you</u> trust yourself to figure things out, face challenges, and reach your goals

Here's why they all matter: *Self-love* means caring for yourself in a deep, respectful way—not just when you're winning, but even when you're struggling. And to really practice self-love, you need all three:

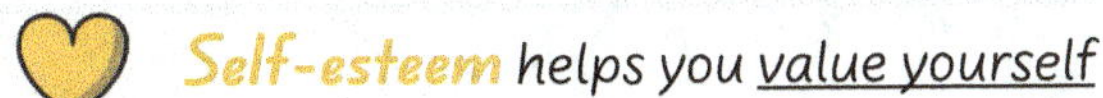 *Self-esteem* helps you <u>value yourself</u>

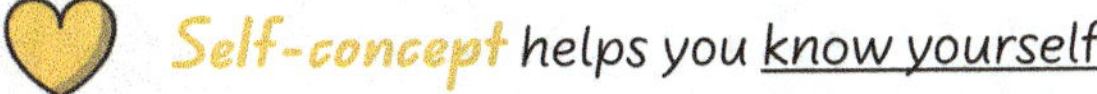 *Self-concept* helps you <u>know yourself</u>

 *Self-efficacy* helps you <u>trust yourself</u>

When these three are strong, self-love becomes something you live, not just a good idea you hear about.

Now, real talk: Your self-esteem, self-concept, and self-efficacy aren't only shaped by what's happening inside you. They're also affected by the world around you, including your family, culture, community, and all the "-isms" *(like racism, sexism, homophobia, ableism, etc.). So if you've ever struggled to feel good about yourself, <u>it's not just you</u>. There are real forces at play that can make it harder.*

When you're feeling good about yourself and your abilities, you might notice:

 You try new things without totally freaking out

 You smile easily and naturally

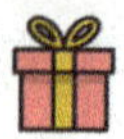 You accept compliments and even believe them!

 You look at challenges and think, <u>I can figure this out</u>

 You carry yourself with quiet confidence

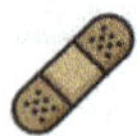 You see mistakes as temporary setbacks, not proof that you're a failure

But when you're struggling with low self-esteem, it might show up like this:

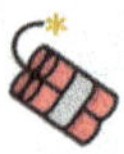 You get discouraged or frustrated really easily

 You feel weird or uncomfortable when someone compliments you

 You procrastinate because you're scared you'll mess up

 You hide from others or isolate yourself

 You avoid trying new things because you think you'll fail

 You constantly second-guess yourself

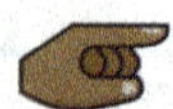 You blame yourself for things that aren't even your fault

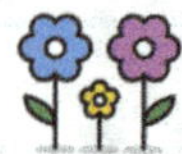 You think everyone else is just <u>better</u> than you

It's really important to remember: Yes, we are responsible for taking care of ourselves and building ourselves up—<u>but</u> we also have to recognize how the outside world affects us. Those -isms we talked about? They show up in small but powerful ways every day. Those little slights, dismissals, or insults? They're called <u>microaggressions</u>—a term created by Dr. Chester Pierce, a Black Caribbean psychiatrist—and they can seriously hurt our self-concept and chip away at how we see ourselves over time.

This is why practicing self-love is such powerful work, especially if you have marginalized identities. Self-love isn't selfish. It's survival. It's resistance. It's choosing to believe in your worth even when the world tries to make you forget it. And every step you take toward loving yourself, even the tiniest one, matters.

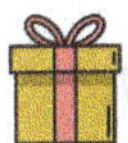 JOURNAL PROMPT

When you think about yourself, what are the first words that pop into your mind? Are they kind, critical, proud, curious? What would it feel like to talk to yourself with the same respect and encouragement you would give someone you care about?

If you had to describe who you are without mentioning your grades, your achievements, or how you look, what would you say? What parts of yourself do you want to know better and celebrate more?

Think of a time when you overcame something hard—even if it felt small. What strengths helped you get through it? How would it feel to trust those strengths the next time you face something challenging?

MINDSET 6

When Hurting Yourself Feels Like the Only Way

Sometimes, when people struggle with how they see themselves—when self-esteem feels low, or when believing in their own strength feels impossible—it can lead to deep emotional pain. One way that some people try to cope with this pain is through something called **non-suicidal self-injury**, or **NSSI**. Let's talk about what that means, and why understanding it with compassion is so important.

NSSI occurs when someone hurts themselves on purpose, *not* because they want to die, but because they're trying to deal with emotional pain. Cutting, pinching, biting, or banging your head against a wall—these are all ways NSSI can show up. Sometimes people self-harm to punish themselves for feeling like they're "too much" or "not enough." More often, it's because physical pain feels easier to handle than emotional pain. For a few moments, it can seem like a release. But that relief is temporary; it doesn't heal the deeper hurt underneath.

If you've ever struggled with this, you are not alone.

In research from The AAKOMA Project, almost 34% (33.8%) of diverse young people reported that they have engaged in NSSI. That's *one in three*—way more common than most people realize.[19]

While it's really important to talk about self-harm honestly, it's just as important to talk about the struggles underneath it—especially struggles with self-concept (how you see yourself) and self-esteem (how you feel about yourself). If you've ever felt like you don't fit in, or worried you'll always be alone, you're not weird—you're human. These feelings are

19. Breland-Noble, A., The AAKOMA Project, and C. A. Harb. *State of Mental Health of Youth and Young Adults of Color,* Full Report. 2025.

especially common during middle school and junior high, when everyone is trying to figure out who they are and where they belong.

And here's something most people don't tell you: Your self-concept doesn't just start when you're a teenager. It starts way earlier, even before you're born. Scientists call this **biopsychosocial stress**—a fancy term that basically means your emotional, physical, and social experiences (and the experiences of your parents and grandparents) shape you *before* you even take your first breath.

If you've ever heard about how maternal and infant health outcomes are worse for Black women and babies, that's a real example of how society's inequalities can impact your health before you've even taken your first breath. Your ancestors' experiences, and the stress they carried, can leave a mark. Then, once you're here in the world, you're met with even more messages about what people like you are "supposed" to be.

You learn it from history books, TV shows, movies, family stories, and now, more than ever, social media. Think about how often you scroll, hoping to see an influencer who actually looks like you, talks like you, or shares your experiences. According to the SOMHYOC 2025 study, 25–35% of young people said they don't see enough high-profile influencers who represent their background.[20] That lack of representation matters—because when you don't see yourself, it can be harder to believe you matter . . . meaning that you're more likely to deal with the kind of emotional pain that can lead to things like NSSI.

That's the hard news. But there's good news, too: Your self-concept isn't only shaped by negativity. It's shaped by love, by pride, by the people who celebrate you. Maybe it's your lola, abuela, or pop-pop telling you how much you remind them of your parent when they were young. Maybe it's your friends hyping you up with a "slayyyyyy" when you walk into school looking incredible. Maybe it's a mentor or teacher telling you how proud they are of the amazing person you're becoming.

The big takeaway here is this: You deserve to be surrounded by people and environments that remind you of your worth. You deserve messaging that tells you:

- You are valuable.
- You come from strength.
- You can create a life that feels good and true to who *you* are.

---

20. Breland-Noble, A., The AAKOMA Project, and C. A. Harb. *State of Mental Health of Youth and Young Adults of Color*, Full Report. 2025.

When you have a strong, healthy self-concept, you don't have to do everything alone—but you *do* believe in your ability to grow, heal, and reach for your dreams. Self-love means recognizing that you are already enough—even when you're still becoming. And when you choose to protect and nurture that self-love, you're choosing to invest in the incredible person you already are, and the even more powerful person you're becoming.

When Food Becomes the Fight: Dealing with Eating Disorders

Let's talk about something that's not always easy to see—especially when we're having a tough time. It's the fact that you *are* strong, valuable, and capable, even when it doesn't feel that way (which I've reminded you of multiple times throughout this book, on purpose!). When we're struggling, it can be really hard to recognize our own worth. That doesn't mean we've lost it—it just means we might need a little help seeing it again.

And here's something really important: Some things just can't be faced alone. Eating disorders are one of those things. Trying to deal with them in isolation doesn't work. Research shows again and again that having people around you who understand and support you is one of the most important parts of recovery.

You might be wondering—why bring that up here? Because disordered eating is a serious issue that a lot of young people face, and it deserves our attention. It's not just "skipping a few meals" or "overeating once in a while." It's a pattern of thinking and behavior that revolves around food, control, and often, pain.

There are a few main types—like binge eating (eating a lot in one sitting and feeling out of control), or restrictive eating (barely eating or obsessing over what you can and can't eat). But here's something a lot of people don't talk about: Eating disorders can affect *anyone*. Nearly 30 million people in the U.S. and 78 million worldwide are impacted.[21, 22] And here's another truth: Eating disorders don't look the same for everyone.

---

21. Harvard T.H. Chan School of Public Health. *Report: Economic Costs of Eating Disorders.* Strategic Training Initiative for the Prevention of Eating Disorders (STRIPED), n.d. https://hsph.harvard.edu/research/eating-disorders-striped/research-reports/economic-costs-eating-disorders/.
22. National Eating Disorders Association. "General Eating Disorder Statistics." National Eating Disorders Association, n.d. https://www.nationaleatingdisorders.org/statistics/#general-eating-disorder-statistics.

The pressures are different, depending on who you are. For example, White girls often face pressure to look a certain way because of media's obsession with thinness. But for Girls of Color, the problem often runs even deeper—systemic racism, cultural invisibility, and unfair expectations all play a role. For example, organizations like Project HEAL and the National Eating Disorders Association teach us that thin body ideals for White girls heavily influence the development of disordered eating, while among Girls of Color, systemic racism is a significant influence on the development of disordered eating.

Unfortunately, too many doctors and therapists aren't trained to recognize disordered eating in boys or Girls of Color. That means too many young people don't get the help they need. That's why it's so important that *you* know this. Awareness is the first step toward change—whether you're struggling yourself or trying to support someone else.

At the end of the day, eating disorders aren't really about food. They're often about control—trying to find *some* way to feel powerful when everything else in life feels messy, overwhelming, or out of your hands. Controlling what you eat, or don't eat, can start to feel like the only thing you *can* control. But over time, that control starts to control you. That's why understanding eating struggles is so connected to learning self-love. Because real self-love isn't just about liking how you look—it's about choosing to care for yourself even when you feel like you don't deserve it. It's about learning that you don't have to hurt your body to feel in charge of your life. You don't have to earn your worth through pain. You already matter. And healing starts when you begin to believe that.

Use the QR code here to learn more about the basic signs and symptoms of eating disorders, and to find some supportive resources.

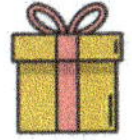 ## JOURNAL PROMPT

Think about a time when you hurt yourself—physically, emotionally, or by denying yourself care or kindness. What were you feeling in that moment? What did you need that maybe you didn't know how to ask for?

Now, imagine that a younger version of you—someone tender and vulnerable—is living through that moment. What would you want them to hear? What kind of love or protection would you offer?

Write a letter to that version of you. No judgment. Just honesty, compassion, and the beginning of a different kind of story.

I Know I'm a Gift, but I Don't Always Feel It—How Do I Help Myself?

There are so many messages out there trying to convince you that you're not good enough. They come from social media, school, sometimes even family or friends, and definitely from society at large. And when you're getting hit with those messages over and over, it can mess with your sense of who you are. That's why practicing self-love isn't just a feel-good idea— it's survival. But to really love ourselves, we have to get honest about what's in the way.

We've already talked about some of the major things that can mess with how you see yourself—like dealing with trauma, identity-based bullying, feeling unseen or misunderstood, or just surviving in a world that doesn't always feel built for you (because, spoiler, it wasn't). If you've experienced any of that, you're not alone—and you deserve tools that actually help. So keep reading. Because the next part is about *you* taking your power back.

If you've ever had to walk through life with a marginalized identity— whether that's about race, gender, sexuality, disability, mental health, or anything else—you already know what it feels like to be misjudged. People might treat you like you're too much, not enough, or just flat-out invisible. It's exhausting. As the legendary Toni Morrison said, that's the whole point of racism and discrimination: to distract you. To throw you off your game. But you can learn to spot those distractions for what they are. And once you can name them, you can resist them.

So let's talk about **racial trauma** and **racial fatigue**. The AAKOMA Project defines racial trauma as the mental and emotional injury caused by encounters with racism, racial bias, racial/ethnic discrimination, and racial hate crimes. We define racial fatigue as the weight of the unseen battles that People of Color face every day related to race, including the heaviness of the weight of racism and discrimination, as well as the tiredness that comes from carrying the burden of dealing with racism and discrimination daily.

This isn't about one big event. This is about the everyday grind—the microaggressions, the headlines, the silence in classrooms, the jokes that aren't funny, the constant pressure to "prove" yourself. Some older generations may brush it off, say it's just part of life. But we name it trauma because that's what it is. And you can't heal something you refuse to name.

This doesn't only apply to race. There are other types of identity-based trauma, too. Bias shows up in different ways—related to your gender, your sexuality, where your family comes from, whether or not you speak English at home, your body, your abilities. And the more identities you hold that get overlooked or disrespected in this world, the more likely it is that your emotional health takes a hit.

So how do you take care of yourself in a world that sometimes tries to wear you down?

Let's break it down:

1. **Learn your history.** Your story didn't start with you. There's strength in the people who came before you—your ancestors, your elders, your cultural traditions. Tapping into that legacy can make you feel less alone and remind you that you're part of something bigger.

2. **Find inspiring role models.** Look for people who light you up—whether it's someone at school, a family member, a mentor, or someone you follow online who speaks truth to power. Let their strength remind you of your own. You don't have to do it all by yourself or reinvent the wheel. We're all here to walk one another home.

3. **Practice self-love again and again.** This is a long-haul journey. It's not about loving yourself perfectly or every second of the day. It's about coming back to kindness, over and over, especially when you're struggling. Think *marathon,* not sprint.

4. **Surround yourself with people who lift you up.** Seriously—check your circle. Who really has your back? Who listens without judging? Who encourages you to be your whole self, not just the version they're comfortable with? Those are the people you keep close. Anyone who drains you? It's OK to set some distance. Pruning your relationships is part of growth.

5. **Use affirmations.** Start your day by saying kind things to yourself—out loud. It may feel weird at first, but it works. Try: "In every moment, I am liberated to choose." That means: *I get to decide how I show up in the world.* Every. Single. Day.

Here's what I want you to really hear: How you feel about yourself is shaped by the world, yes. But it is not *defined* by it. *You* determine your worth. Your value isn't up for debate. And building a strong sense of self starts with turning toward yourself, with love. That's how you learn to spot the people who will really see you—and how you begin to step into your own story, fully.

Everyone's path is different. Honor yours. Trust it. And keep walking forward—even when the world tries to block your way. You're more powerful than you've been taught to believe.

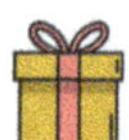 ## JOURNAL PROMPT

Which of the suggestions for helping you see and know yourself as a gift gave you the most peace? Why do you think that is? Which of these strategies can you start incorporating into your life to help you steady yourself when you feel "less than" to remind you that you are so much more than your worst days?

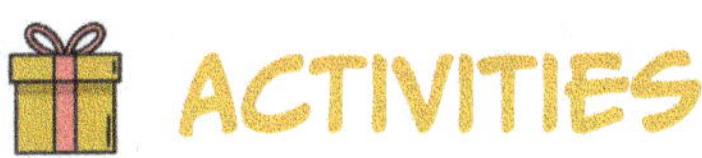

ACTIVITIES

Now that you know something about how we can practice self-love with care and intention, let's practice some new skills.

EASY

A Tiny Pause

For one week, before you reach for your phone in the morning—before the scrolling, the notifications, the flood of everyone else's thoughts—give yourself thirty seconds of silence. No distractions, no noise. Just you, waking up with yourself. You might stare at the ceiling, take a deep breath, stretch your fingers, or let your mind wander. It might feel awkward at first, or even boring. But notice what it's like to *not* hand your attention over right away. At the end of the week, write about it. Did anything shift in how your days began? Did your thoughts feel different when you gave them space before the noise? What surprised you? This tiny pause is a way of reminding yourself: *You come first.*

After this activity, I feel:

MODERATE

The Post-it Oracle

Get a set of multicolored Post-its and a small glass bowl. Use ChatGPT to brainstorm thirty positive adjectives that you think describe you. Write each word down on one Post-it, fold the Post-it in half, and drop it in the bowl. Every day, before you touch your cell or device, find a space to sit quietly for just five minutes. Grab the bowl and set it in front of you. Close your eyes and take a Post-it from the bowl. This is your encouragement for the day. Like Queen Ramonda from *Black Panther* told T'Challa, "Remember who you are."

After this activity, I feel:

HARD

Mental Help

Grab a calendar, grab a device. Set a one-per-week reminder to look for a mental-health professional who fits your needs (use one of the many databases available for this purpose). For a month, take thirty minutes each week to look for a psychotherapist whom you *would* go to if you could. Learn all about them, their approach, and their fees. Do they offer telehealth or not? How many years of experience, specialty areas, etc., do they have? You're only looking and searching for this one month. After the month, you should have a list of providers at the ready in case you ever want to reach out for help to someone you sense would best meet your needs. It takes real power and self-love to identify the help that serves you best.

After this activity, I feel:

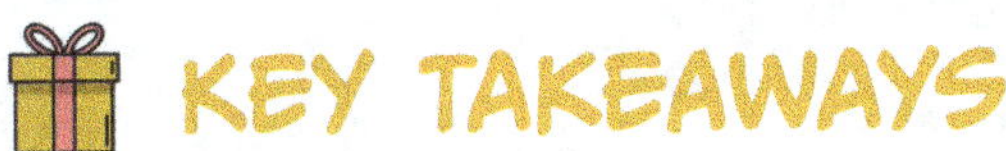 # KEY TAKEAWAYS

Congrats! You made it to the end of Mindset 6: You Are a Gift! Have you learned anything you want to incorporate into your daily routine? Is there anything in this section you want to shout from the rooftops about? Maybe you've learned something you can share with your friends or parents/caregivers to help them. Make a note of your key takeaways (including the ones you'd like to share with others) and write them below:

MINDSET 6

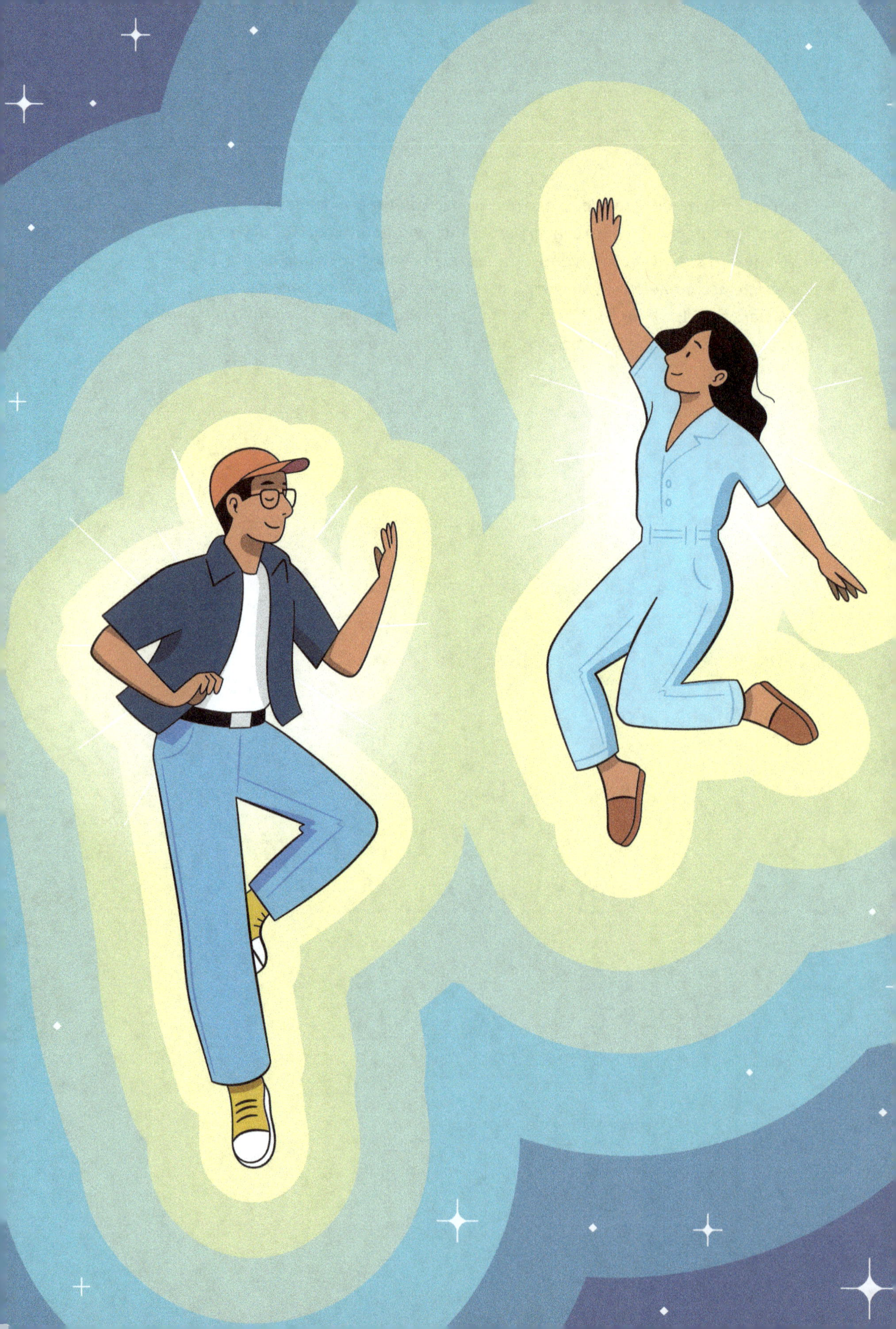

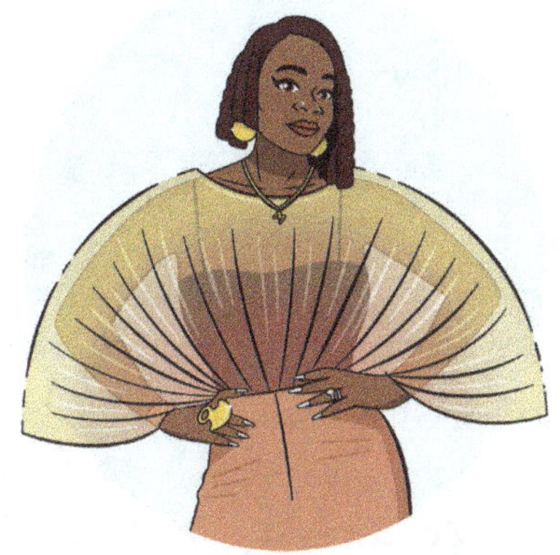

Love Inside,
Love Outside

You already know you don't have to earn the right to be treated with dignity. That's your birthright. But in a world that often tries to shrink or silence young people—especially if you're queer, trans, a Person of Color, neurodivergent, or just someone who doesn't fit the mold—it's easy to believe that invisibility is safer. That staying quiet is survival. And sometimes it *is*. But over time, that quiet can eat away at your sense of worth. That's why self-love, as you learned in Mindset 6, isn't just personal—it's revolutionary. When you start honoring yourself, you begin to attract and build relationships where you're celebrated, not just tolerated. And when we gather in that kind of love? That's when communities come alive.

You don't have to wait until you're older, richer, or more "together" to make a difference. Start with your group chat, your lunch table, your little sibling. What does it look like to show up with respect, with honesty, with care? What does it feel like to know you helped someone else feel seen, even if just for a moment? These small acts aren't small. They're seeds. And when enough of us plant them, we grow something big—a world where everyone gets to belong. That's the kind of world you're already helping to build, just by being here.

By the end of this section, you will know more about:

- What it looks like to diligently practice self-love, especially when life knocks you down
- How to love and respect yourself and others
- How to build positive community that honors you and the person you want to be

Let's Get Started

Back when I was a professor, I had a meeting with someone who was supposed to be my mentor. She was a woman like me—but she wasn't a Woman of Color. I'd recently found out that I was being underpaid compared to others doing the same job, and I had the receipts to prove it. Since she'd actually recruited me for the role and had been in the field a lot longer, I figured she'd want to help me figure out what to do. So during one of our regular check-ins, I brought it up—calmly, clearly. I told her I thought I deserved a salary adjustment (not even a raise, just to be paid fairly). Her response? She looked me dead in the eye and said, "Alfiee, you didn't come here to get rich."

That moment stung. Not just because I felt dismissed as a mentee, but because I'd hoped she might get it—as a fellow woman, as someone who knew what it was like to be overlooked. But instead, it felt like she was telling me to stay quiet, be grateful, and accept less.

My best guess? Maybe she thought I was being too bold for speaking up. Maybe she felt like I was throwing shade on her career by saying this place wasn't it for me. I'll never know exactly what she was thinking, but I do know that was the moment I realized this job wasn't my home.

It took me a year and a half to make a plan and leave—but I did it. I walked away and chose to believe in a future where I didn't have to shrink to fit in. A future where I could find or build a community that valued me the same way I had finally started to value myself. A future where I could be part of a movement of people working to mutually lift up and empower one another.

And where did I find this community after years of longing for it? *I built it myself,* and you know it as The AAKOMA Project 501(c)(3) nonprofit, where, "We envision a world where EVERY child, teen, and young adult (inclusive of all points of diversity) feels the freedom to live unapologetically and authentically within an environment that allows them to rise and thrive."

I built AAKOMA because I needed AAKOMA. I needed a work environment free from the toxicity of systemic racism, sexism, homophobia, xenophobia, socioeconomic bias, and so many other forms of discrimination. I needed a place where my motives for wanting to uplift myself (and those who have been marginalized) were not questioned or considered far-fetched. A place where I could get up in the morning excited to go to work, and where I knew that I could live out my purpose free from impediments.

I did not find that place until I made that place.

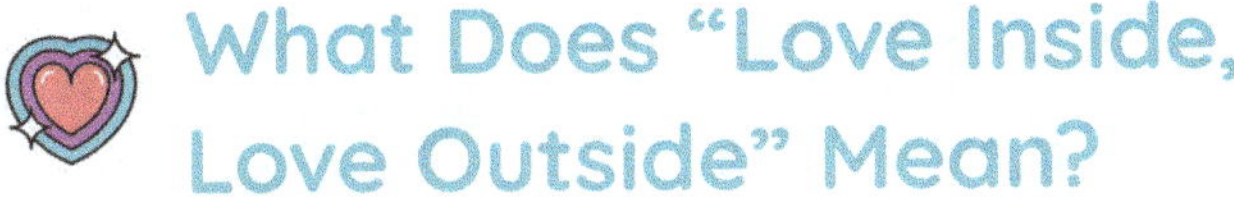 What Does "Love Inside, Love Outside" Mean?

Love is real. It's not just some abstract idea from a movie or a sappy quote on Instagram—it's authentic, active, and when it's right, it feels amazing. Whether it's love for your best friends, your family, your soulmate, or even just the way your community shows up for you, love is what fills you up, fuels you, and reminds you that you matter.

Real love isn't about perfection; it's about being seen, valued, and respected. That's why I say love is *active*. It's something you *do*—not just something you say. You have to *practice* it, both toward yourself and toward others. Love doesn't live in theory—it lives in actions, in choices, in showing up.

When you're true to yourself, when you act in line with your own values, and when you take the time to figure out what actually makes you *you*, you're practicing self-love. We talked about this back in Mindset 6: Self-love and self-respect are deeply connected. It's tough to love someone you don't respect, and it's often hard to respect someone you don't love—even if that love is quiet, distant, or just appreciation for what they bring out in you. So let's build on that. There are some key things to remember about actively practicing self-love—and it starts with honoring your own needs, being kind to yourself when it's hardest, and making space for your truth, even when others don't fully get it yet.

Now, when we turn that love outward, what does that look like? That's where our relationships come in—whether it's with friends, romantic partners, classmates, or family. You probably learned the golden rule when you were a little kid: *Treat others the way you want to be treated.* But that's only part of the picture. Because what makes *you* feel good (say, a giant bear hug every time you see someone) might make someone else super uncomfortable.

So what if we flip it a little? It's not about copying how *you* want to be loved—it's about showing others the same level of care and respect you'd want in a way they can actually receive it. That's the deeper truth behind the golden rule. It's not about assuming, it's about attuning. That's how we build trust, build love, and build communities that feel like home—for everyone.

Signs and Symptoms of Love Inside, Love Outside

So what does love _actually_ look like in action? I'm glad you asked. Here are a few simple, powerful ways we practice love for our full selves:

 We speak kind words to ourselves—even when no one else is watching

 We forgive our mistakes and treat them as opportunities to grow, not reasons to spiral

 We stop comparing ourselves to others—your journey is yours, and that's your magic

 We hype ourselves up daily—a pep talk in the mirror counts, FYI

 We spend quiet time reflecting on what we've done well, not just what we need to fix

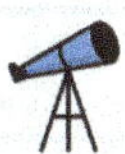 We dream and plan for our future, no matter how far off it seems

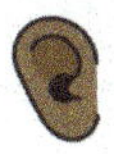 We listen to our inner voice—that gut feeling that knows what's right for us

And here's how we show love to the people around us—the friends, family, partners, and communities we care about:

 Transparent communication—we say what we mean and listen when others do, too

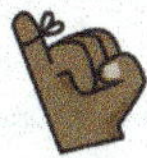 Accountability—we own our actions, even when it's hard

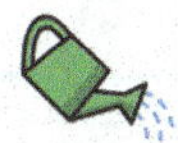 Responsibility—we show up and follow through

 Kindness—we lead with care, not just vibes

 Trustworthiness—we keep it real and keep our promises

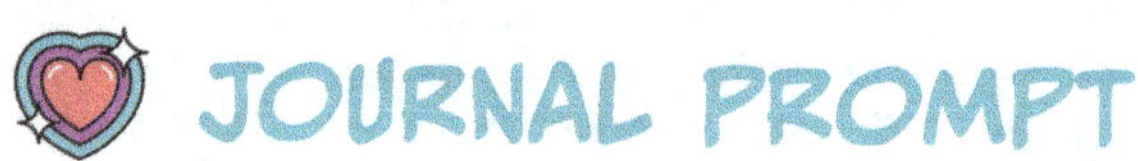

JOURNAL PROMPT

Choose one way you show love to yourself and one way you show love to someone else from the lists above. Reflect on how each one has shown up in your life recently. What helped you practice that kind of love—or what held you back? How did it impact your sense of connection, safety, or trust with yourself and with others? Then imagine: What would your relationships look like if both kinds of love—inner and outer—were active, steady, and real every day? What would change? What would feel more possible?

Loving and Respecting Ourselves and Others

Once we start getting the hang of self-love and self-respect—and yeah, that's an ongoing process, not a one-time "I got it!" moment—we can begin to shift our focus toward how we show up with others. That's what the second half of Mindset 7 is all about: *love outside.*

Have you ever found yourself struggling in a relationship? And I don't just mean a romantic one—this could be with a friend, a classmate, someone you work with, even a family member. When we're babies, our relationships are pretty simple—we depend on a small circle of people to care for us. But as we grow and move through the world, we meet more people and form all kinds of new relationships. That can be exciting, sure, but it can also get messy—especially when there's conflict, misunderstanding, bullying, or rejection.

Here's something to think about: A lot of the hurtful stuff people do comes from their *own* wounds. I see conflict and polarization as downstream effects of people not feeling loved, safe, or seen enough. And that's exactly why self-love matters so much. The tools we use to care for *ourselves*—like communicating honestly, being accountable, and keeping our word—can help prevent conflict with *others*. That's the power of love inside and love outside working together.

Right now, our world is full of division. You see it every day—in global wars, climate change denial, attacks on trans youth, racist violence, police brutality, and more. That polarization spills into our daily lives too, giving people a kind of permission to act in harmful ways—bullying others, making threats, starting conflict. It's not just out there on the news; it's happening online, in schools, in DMs. In our 2025 SOMHYOC study, 30% of diverse teens and young adults said they'd been threatened online about their race or ethnicity, and 31% said they'd been excluded online for the same reason.[23]

Maybe that's even happened to you. Maybe someone you trusted suddenly flipped the script and started treating you harshly or unfairly. If it has—I'm so sorry. That kind of betrayal hurts deeply. I've felt it too. And I want to offer you some tools that might help.

When trust gets broken, especially by someone you care about, it can feel like the *last* moment you'd want to think about love. But actually, that's *exactly* when Mindset 7—Love Inside, Love Outside—becomes most powerful. Here's what you can try:

- **Acknowledge the hurt**—remember that naming what's real flames blame and shame.
- **Name the hurt in detail**—don't skip over it. Be honest about what happened.

23. Breland-Noble, A., The AAKOMA Project, and C. A. Harb. *State of Mental Health of Youth and Young Adults of Color,* Full Report. 2025.

- **Understand why it hurt you**—what value or boundary got crossed?
- **Decide what healing looks like**—is it confronting the person (if it feels physically and emotionally safe)? Or is it creating space and healing on your own, away from them?

Now you might be thinking: *OK,* but *they* hurt me. *Why should I be the one doing all this emotional work?* And you know what? Fair question. You don't *have* to. You're not obligated to fix things that weren't your fault. But here's the thing: your healing matters more than their apology. You're doing this for *you.* Because *you* deserve peace. *You* deserve to start from a place of love inside, always.

That's why I believe in self-care as more than bubble baths and playlists (though those can help too). Self-care is about reclaiming your story and your strength. It's why I wrote this book—because you deserve healing. You

deserve relationships that feel safe and real. And who knows? As you walk your own path to healing, you might just light the way for someone else to begin theirs. That's love outside in action.

Check out the following video about the four steps of self-care I mentioned above by using the QR code here.

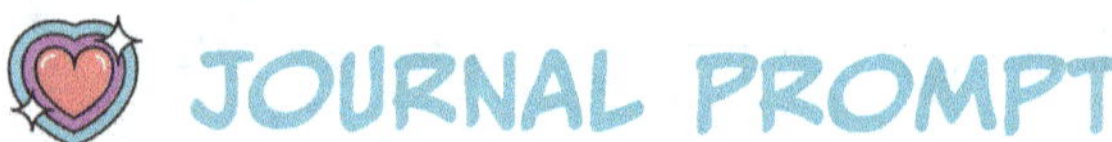

💗 JOURNAL PROMPT

Think about a time when you were hurt, misunderstood, or excluded in a relationship. How did you respond—and how did it feel to respond that way? Now, looking back with everything you've learned in this book, ask yourself: What would it have looked like to stay in solidarity with yourself in that moment? What tools—like self-respect, clear communication, boundaries, or reflection—could have helped you move through that experience with more strength and self-love?

Then, write about what inner fortitude means to you. How do you stay rooted in your values even when you're tested? What does it mean to act with integrity in your relationships, without abandoning yourself? Finish by imagining what it would feel like to move through the world knowing that you have your own back—consistently, lovingly, and without apology.

____

____

____

____

____

____

____

____

I Know About "Love Inside, Love Outside," but How Do I Apply It to Myself?

I recently watched a movie called *Sinners*, directed by Ryan Coogler and starring Michael B. Jordan, and let me tell you, it hit *hard*. One of the biggest themes in the film is community—what it means to find it, build it, protect it, and keep it alive. For folks from diverse backgrounds, community isn't just a "nice-to-have." It's essential. It's a mirror that reflects back your worth, your beauty, your strength, and all the possibilities your life holds.

You deserve to find your people. Because when you do, it feels like coming home. And we all need a home base—somewhere we're accepted exactly as we are. So as you start to seek or build that kind of community, here are a few powerful questions to ask yourself:

- *What does a positive community actually look like?*
- *How do I build that kind of community?*
- *Who feels aligned enough to be in community with me?*
- *And when is it time to invite someone out of my community with love and clarity?*

Reflecting on these questions helps you sharpen your understanding of *love outside*—the second half of Mindset 7. You start to figure out where to go when you need support and how to show up in ways that support others. Sometimes, the most meaningful thing you can offer someone in your circle isn't a solution—it's presence. It's sitting with them, distraction-free, listening deeply. Other times, it's a kind word, a gentle check-in, or some real talk (if they ask for it). Those small acts? They build trust. They build alliance.

That's what love outside is all about: creating relationships where everyone gets to be real, where nobody has to shrink. And guess what? When you show up like that for others, you raise the standard—not just for how you want to be treated, but for how your whole community learns to love. This kind of leadership isn't loud or flashy, but it's transformational. It even helps bridge gaps between generations—like when your Gen X or Millennial parents or your Boomer grandparents just don't get your worldview. Love inside, love outside means honoring the connection while standing firm in your truth.

So how do you actually *practice* love inside and love outside in your daily life? Here are five powerful tools to help you show up for yourself *and* others:

1. **Be honest with yourself and others.** Telling the truth—especially when it's uncomfortable—is a major act of love. It shows self-respect and builds real trust with others. Honesty doesn't mean being harsh; it means being clear, kind, and grounded in your values.

2. **Learn the art of repair.** Messing up is part of being human. What matters is how you come back from it. When you hurt someone (even unintentionally), take responsibility, offer a sincere apology, and ask how you can make things right. Repair is how relationships grow stronger, not weaker.

3. **Hold yourself and others accountable.** Accountability isn't about being perfect or policing people—it's about making sure your actions line up with your values. It means you're willing to own your impact and make things right when harm is caused. When you hold yourself accountable, you're showing love inside. When you hold others accountable with care and clarity, you're practicing love outside. For example, say you

laughed along with a joke that put someone down, and later it doesn't sit right with you. You go back and say, "I shouldn't have laughed—I messed up, and I want to be better than that." That's accountability in action. Now imagine a friend says something harmful and brushes it off like it's no big deal. You don't have to cancel them, but you also don't pretend it didn't happen. You might say, "That wasn't OK, and I need you to hear that. I care about you, which is why I'm speaking up." You're not letting harm slide—but you're also giving space for responsibility and growth. That's how strong communities are built.

4. **Be present when others are struggling.** Sometimes, the best way to show love is just to *listen*. No fixing, no advice—just presence. Putting your phone down, making eye contact, and saying "I'm here for you" goes a long way.

5. **Stay grounded in your truth.** Whether you're dealing with peer pressure or family friction, love inside means knowing what matters to *you*—and staying rooted in it. Love outside means offering that same respect to others, even when you disagree. This is an important one, so let me offer an example. Let's say you're in a family conversation and someone makes a comment that feels dismissive of your identity or beliefs. Love inside means you don't shrink or stay silent just to keep the peace—you take a breath, stay grounded, and say, "That actually doesn't sit right with me, and I want to explain why." You're honoring your values and standing in your truth. Love outside doesn't mean excusing harmful behavior—but it does mean addressing it in a way that invites growth. Instead of just canceling the person or blowing up, you might say, "I care about this relationship, which is why I need to speak up. I know we see things differently, but this matters to me." That way, you're still holding a boundary while creating the possibility for real change.

You have the tools now. You've been building them throughout this book. Use them to empower yourself—and to help shape communities where everyone gets to be free, loved, and whole. Starting with you.

💗 JOURNAL PROMPT

Which of the suggestions for helping yourself lit you up the most? Why? Which of the strategies can you start incorporating into your life to strengthen your love inside—and remind yourself of your worth—so you can show up with confidence, even on the hard days, and offer that same love and steadiness to others?

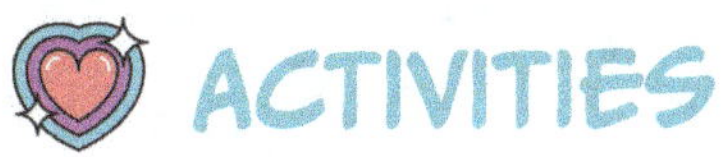 # ACTIVITIES

Now that you know something about how we can practice self-love with care and intention, let's practice some new skills.

EASY

"I Am" Statement

What do you stand for? What do you believe in when no one's looking? What qualities feel true to you—even on the tough days?

Take a moment and create your own "I am" statement—a list of words or phrases that describe your core values and your inner strength. This isn't about how others see you—it's about how you choose to see yourself.

Here's an example to get you started: *I am grounded. I am honest. I am kind to myself. I am loyal to my people. I am creative, thoughtful, and strong— even when I feel shaky. I am becoming exactly who I'm meant to be.*

Now it's your turn. Write it like you mean it. Let it be your mirror, your anchor, your reminder. Stick it on your wall, your phone, your mirror—wherever you need to see it most. Let this be your declaration of love inside.

After this activity, I feel:

MODERATE

A Week of Mindfulness

For the next seven days, take a few minutes each day to check out my **Monday Mindfulness** videos (QR code). These are short, calming, real-talk moments to help you slow down, breathe, and reconnect with yourself—especially when life feels loud or heavy.

Use this time to check in with your love inside. You don't need to "clear your mind" or sit a certain way—just show up as you are. Notice how you feel before and after. Keep a little journal or voice note each day if that helps. By the end of the week, see what's shifted. Even small moments of calm can change everything.

After this activity, I feel:

HARD

Mental-Health Meetup

Find a safe, trusted in-person event happening near you—a youth meetup, club gathering, mental-health event, or community circle. If you're under eighteen, have a parent or guardian check it out with you to make sure it's safe. Then grab a friend (or two!) and go together.

Not sure where to start? Try a mental health-themed volunteer activity—like joining a fundraising walk, helping out at a mental-health fair, or signing up for your school's mental-health or wellness club. Just try it once and see how it feels to be part of something bigger than yourself—something good. Being in community with people who care can remind you that you're not alone, and that you have something powerful to offer the world. That's love outside in action.

After this activity, I feel:

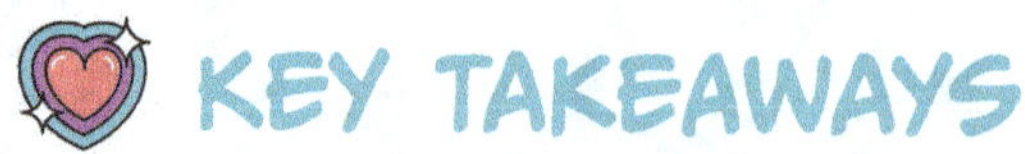 # KEY TAKEAWAYS

Congrats! You made it to the end of Mindset 7: Love Inside, Love Outside. Have you learned anything you want to incorporate into your daily routine? Is there anything in this section you want to shout from the rooftops about? Maybe you've learned something you can share with your friends or parents/caregivers to help them. Make a note of your key takeaways (including the ones you'd like to share with others) and write them below:

Sending You on Your Way with Lots of Love and Light

You get to write the ending to this book—just like you get to write your own story. For real. The story that lives inside you—the one that feels honest, deep, and true in your bones—that's the one that should lead the way. You are the architect of your own life. Use this book as a guide to help you trust yourself more, name your journey out loud, and take full ownership of your story.

You're part of a huge, never-ending story—a *collective* story that connects you to so many others. And the fact that you're here, right now, reading these words? That's no accident. You found this book for a reason, and that matters. I hope the tools and ideas in these pages remind you that just by *existing*, you already help shape the world. Just by being here, you make a difference.

This book isn't about fixing you—it's about *equipping* you. No matter where you are right now—resting, resisting, dreaming, grieving, growing, or just doing your best to stay afloat—these seven mindsets are here to help you care for your mind and spirit while showing up for your people and your community.

Let this sink in:

- You have agency.
- You are powerful.
- You are visionary.
- You are courageous—even on the days you don't feel like it.
- You can do hard things.
- You can take up space.
- You can ask for what you need.
- You can offer support to others.
- You can build the kind of community you've always wanted.
- And yes—you can fall apart, and put yourself back together, again and again, without shame.

And just so we're clear: You *will* get tired. That doesn't mean you've failed. That doesn't mean you're weak. It means you're human. I want you to treat this healing journey like a marathon—not a sprint. It takes time. You're learning to notice what your mind, body, and spirit are asking for—and when exhaustion shows up, I hope you listen.

Rest is not a luxury. Rest is not a reward. Rest is your right. Rest is resistance. Rest is radical. Rest is fuel. Let it fuel your joy. Let it bring you clarity. Let it power your dreams and help you move forward. Rest isn't getting in the way of your growth—it's part of the cycle of growth.

So here's my wish for you: Treat yourself like a dormant orchid—waiting, alive, full of possibility—ready to bloom in your own bright, beautiful, natural colors. Think of this book like water and sunlight and fertilizer. Let the words soak in. Use the journal prompts, the activities, and the reflections to nurture your spirit. You are part of nature's rhythm—and yes, you are meant to *bloom*.

Bloom into the version of you that you know, deep down, you're meant to be. Grow into that version slowly, boldly, tenderly—over days, months, and years. Know that your path is *yours*. It doesn't have to look like anyone else's. Move at your own pace. Even when life feels like it's pulling you in a hundred directions—school, family, work, relationships, community—you have the power to pause, shift your perspective, speak life into yourself, rise back up when you feel knocked down, build your crew, fight for justice, *rise* and *thrive*.

You come first. Not because you're selfish. But because you know *you can't pour into others if your cup is empty.*

Here's what I believe: Deep down, you already know how to start caring for your mental health. But we all need reminders. We all need a gentle nudge. So let this be yours: *You deserve care, too.*

I hope you'll let me walk beside you a little longer—offering whatever I can: wisdom, encouragement, maybe a spark of something sacred passed down through our ancestors. Because we come from people who resisted, survived, created beauty in the middle of chaos, and still found ways to thrive. That strength is in *you*, too. It's in your body, your bones, your blood.

Let that remembrance *root* you. Let it lift you. You're part of something *huge*. Something miraculous. Something called *this life*. You've got this. And you are *enough*—just as you are. So allow me to send you off (on your journey to rising and thriving):

Wishing you love, light, and good, culturally relevant science
—Dr. Alfiee

PS The QR code to the right will take you to the "Parents' Corner" on Dr. Alfiee's website—a space full of videos and resources for parents, guardians, and other trusted adults who want to support the young people (ages thirteen to twenty-five) in their lives.

Final Activity: A Love Note Just for You

You've made it to the end of this book—but really, you've just arrived at a new beginning. For this final activity, take some time to write a love letter to yourself. Yes—you. This is your chance to speak directly to the version of you who needs encouragement, compassion, hype, honesty, and care.

There's no wrong way to do this. You can write it as if you're talking to your present self, your past self, or even the future version of you you're becoming. Be real. Be kind. Be gentle. Say what you wish someone had said to you—and say what *you* know you need to hear now. You can look back over some of your journal entries for inspiration, too. You might want to include:

- What you're proud of
- What you've survived
- What you love about your mind, body, and spirit
- What you're still working on (and how you're rooting for yourself anyway)
- What dreams you hope to chase and protect

When you're done, fold up the letter, tuck it somewhere special, or read it aloud to yourself. Let it be a reminder: You are worthy of your own love. Always.

Check out the QR code to the right, where I share a letter of encouraging, loving words that I wrote to myself years ago—and that remain an inspiration to me to this very day.

About the Author

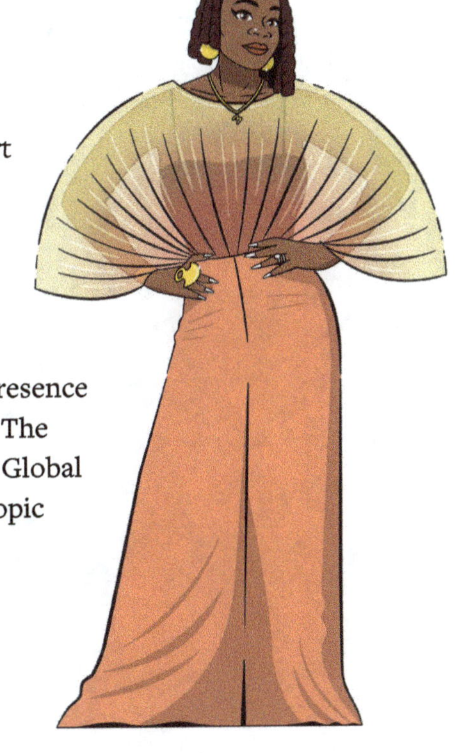

Dr. Alfiee is a mental health trailblazer whose heart and vision have redefined mental health for communities around the world. A graduate of Howard, NYU, the University of Wisconsin-Madison, and the Duke School of Medicine, Dr. Alfiee shares her deep expertise as a liberated psychiatry professor, researcher, in-demand speaker, media presence and founder of the youth mental health nonprofit, The AAKOMA Project. Named a Melinda French Gates Global Leader and entrusted with a $20 million philanthropic fund, her innovative research and programs uplift diverse people everywhere. With her soul-stirring presence, and easy to follow strategies, Dr. Alfiee teaches you how to find and embrace emotional healing, joy, and your authentic self.

Let Dr. Alfiee's spirit and culturally relevant wisdom guide you toward mental wellness, belonging, and boundless possibility.